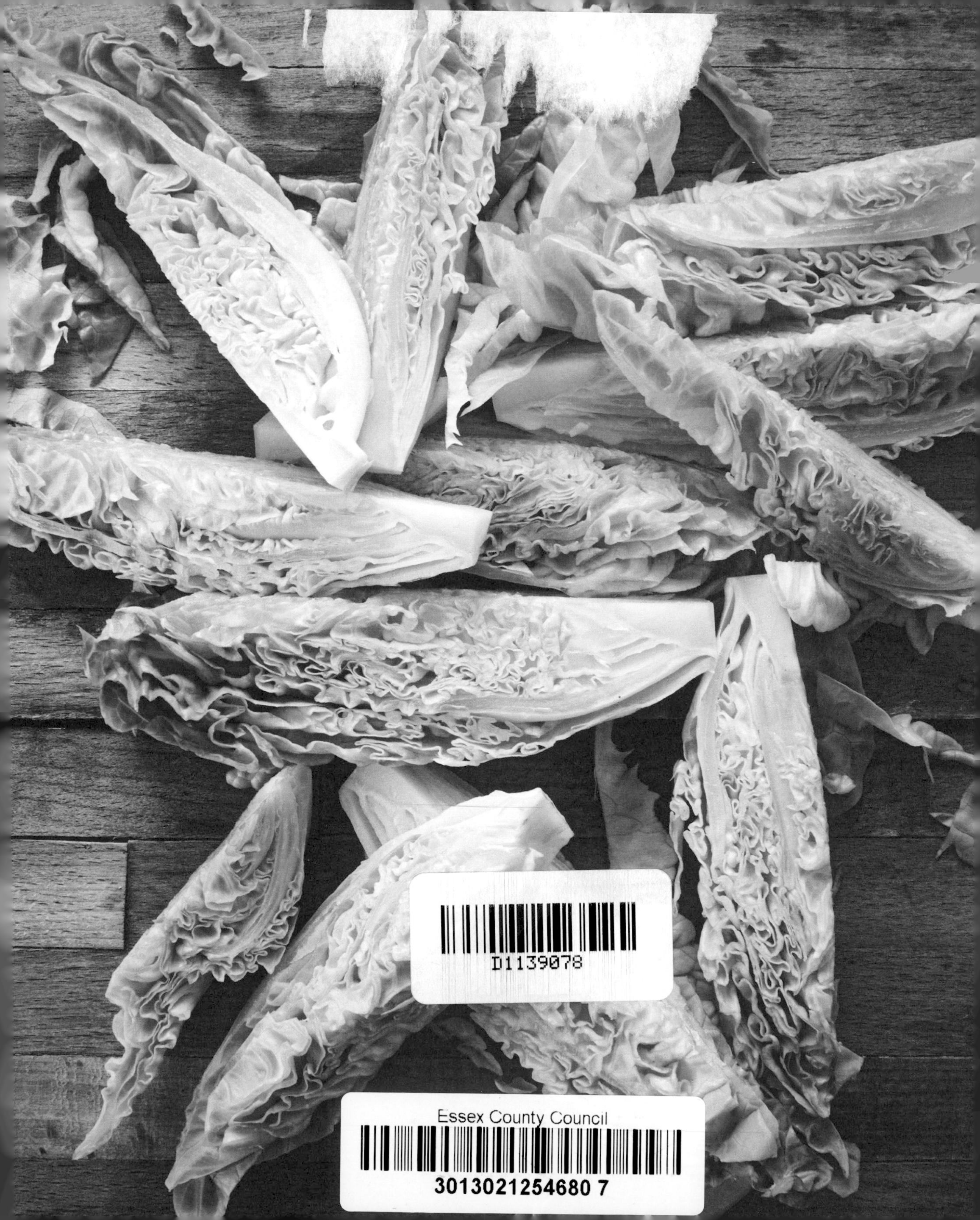

perfectly PALEO

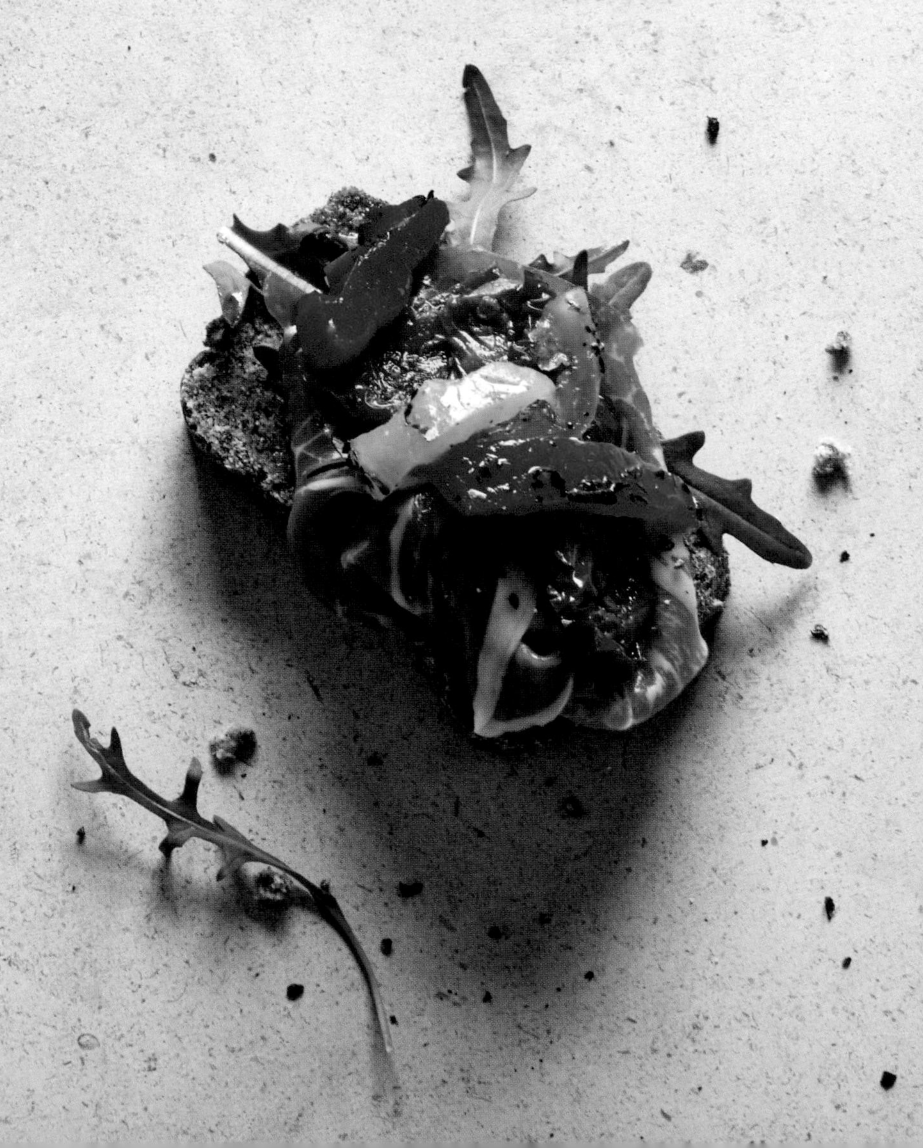

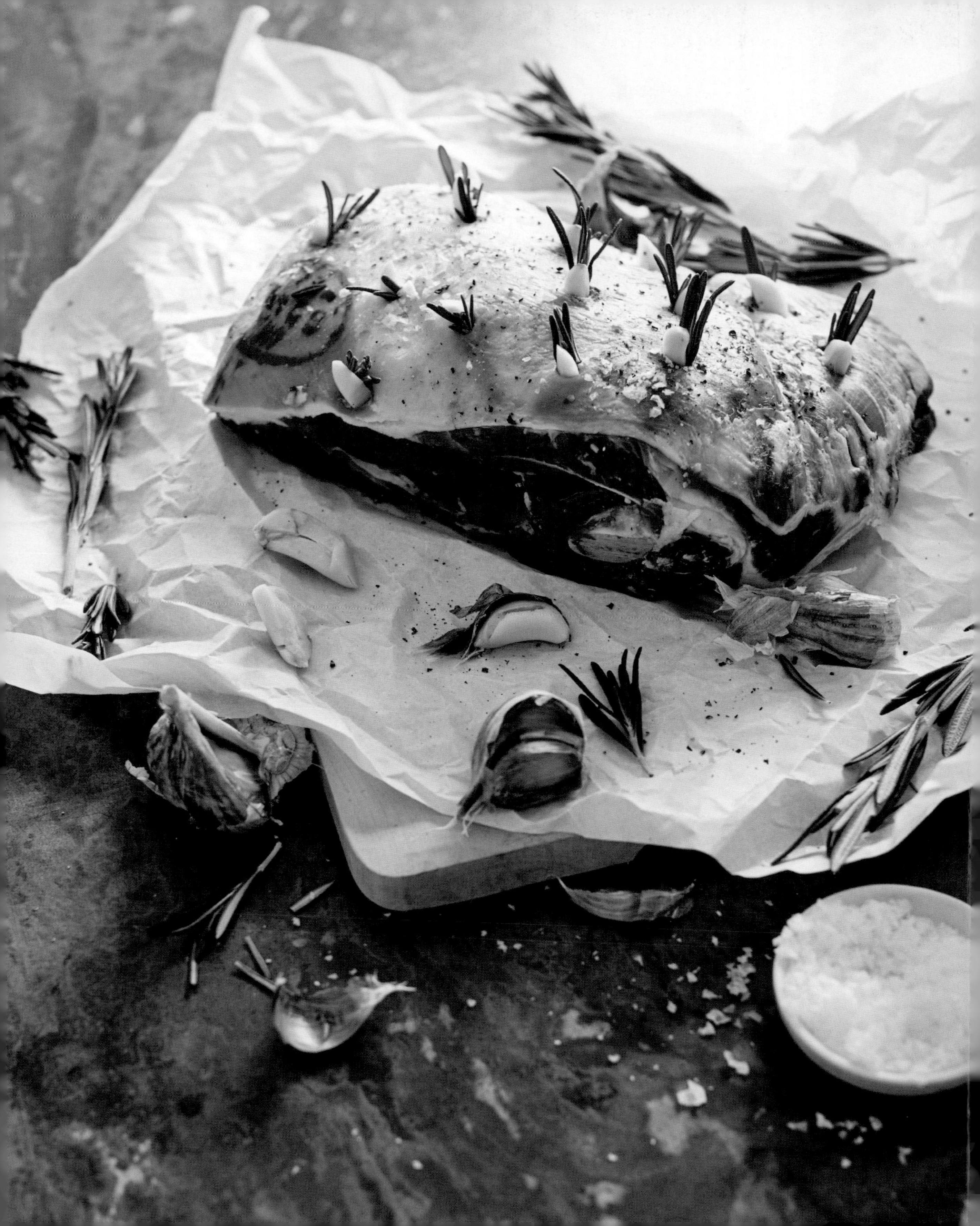

perfectly PALEO

RECIPES FOR CLEAN
EATING ON A PALEO DIET

Rosa Rigby
photography
by Mowie Kay

rps
RYLAND PETERS & SMALL
LONDON • NEW YORK

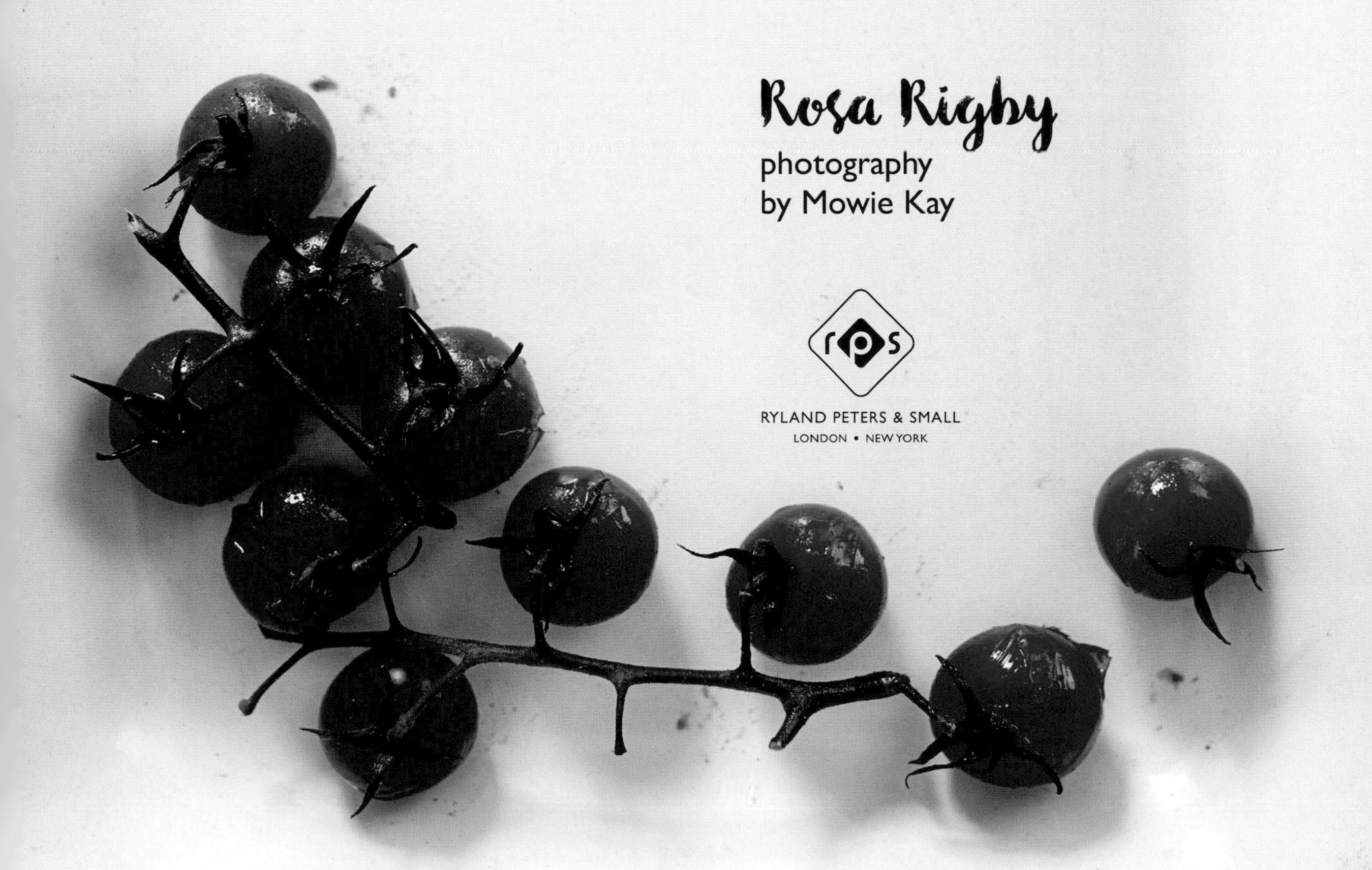

To my family, who have brought me up in an environment of constant appreciation of good produce and home-cooked food. This is really what 'Paleo' is to me.

Senior designer Sonya Nathoo
Commissioning editor Stephanie Milner
Production manager Gordana Simonavic
Art director Leslie Harrington
Editorial director Julia Charles
Publisher Cindy Richards

Food stylist Rachel Wood
Prop stylist Jennifer Kay
Illustrator Lily Rigby
Indexer Hilary Bird

First published in 2016 by
Ryland Peters & Small
20–21 Jockey's Fields,
London WC1R 4BW
and
341 E 116th St,
New York NY 10029

www.rylandpeters.com

10 9 8 7 6 5 4 3 2 1

ISBN: 978-1-84975-770-6

Printed in China

A CIP record for this book is available from the British Library.

US Library of Congress Cataloging-in-Publication Data has been applied for.

Notes

• Both British (Metric) and American (Imperial plus US cups) measurements are included in these recipes for convenience; however it is important to work with one set of measurements and not alternate between the two within a recipe.

• All spoon measurements are level unless otherwise specified.

• All eggs are medium (UK) or large (US), unless specified as large, in which case US extra-large should be used. Uncooked or partially cooked eggs should not be served to the very old, frail, young children, pregnant women or those with compromised immune systems.

• Ovens should be preheated to the specified temperatures. We recommend using an oven thermometer. If using a fan-assisted oven, adjust temperatures according to the manufacturer's instructions.

• When a recipe calls for the grated zest of citrus fruit, buy unwaxed fruit and wash well before using. If you can only find treated fruit, scrub well in warm soapy water before using.

• When a recipe calls for baking powder, bicarbonate of/baking soda and other such standard baking ingredients, check that they are gluten-free in order to follow a Paleo diet.

• To sterilize preserving jars, wash them in hot, soapy water and rinse in boiling water. Place in a large saucepan and cover with hot water. With the saucepan lid on, bring the water to a boil and continue boiling for 15 minutes. Turn off the heat and leave the jars in the hot water until just before they are to be filled. Invert the jars onto a clean kitchen cloth to dry. Sterilize the lids for 5 minutes, by boiling or according to the manufacturer's instructions. Jars should be filled and sealed while they are still hot.

• There are many different brands of nutritional supplements available and each have varying portion recommendations based on their specific blend of ingredients. Standard scoop sizes vary (20–60 g/¾–3 oz.) but most brands usually provide a 1-portion scoop or list the portion size on the packaging. Always refer to the packet instructions when following the recipes within this book. You should consult your physician before beginning a dietary regimen.

• Disclaimer: The views expressed in this book are those of the author but they are general views only and readers are urged to consult a relevant and qualified specialist or physician for individual advice before beginning any dietary regimen. Ryland Peters & Small hereby exclude all liability to the extent permitted by law for any errors or omissions in this book and for any loss, damage or expense (whether direct or indirect) suffered by a third party relying on any information contained in this book.

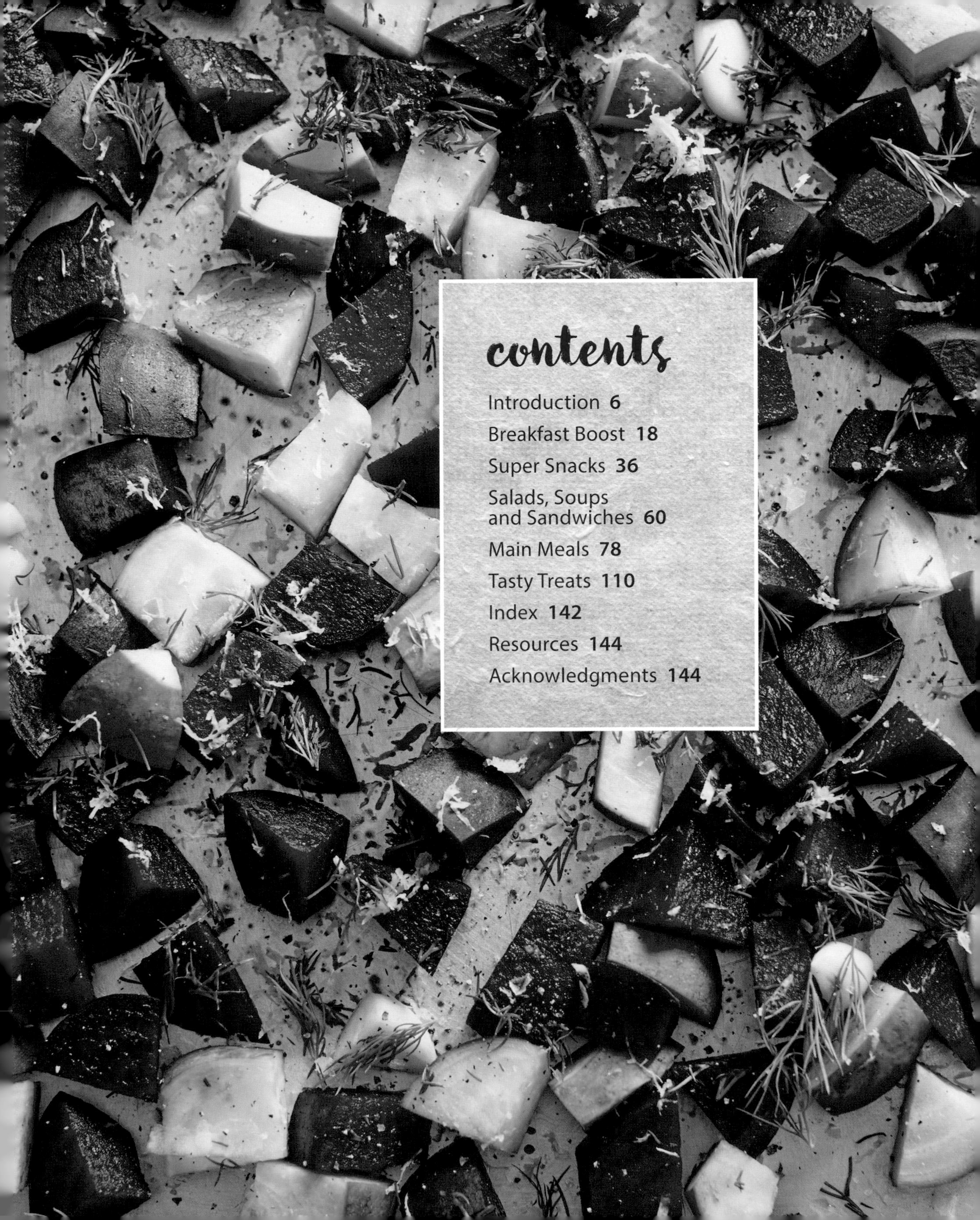

contents

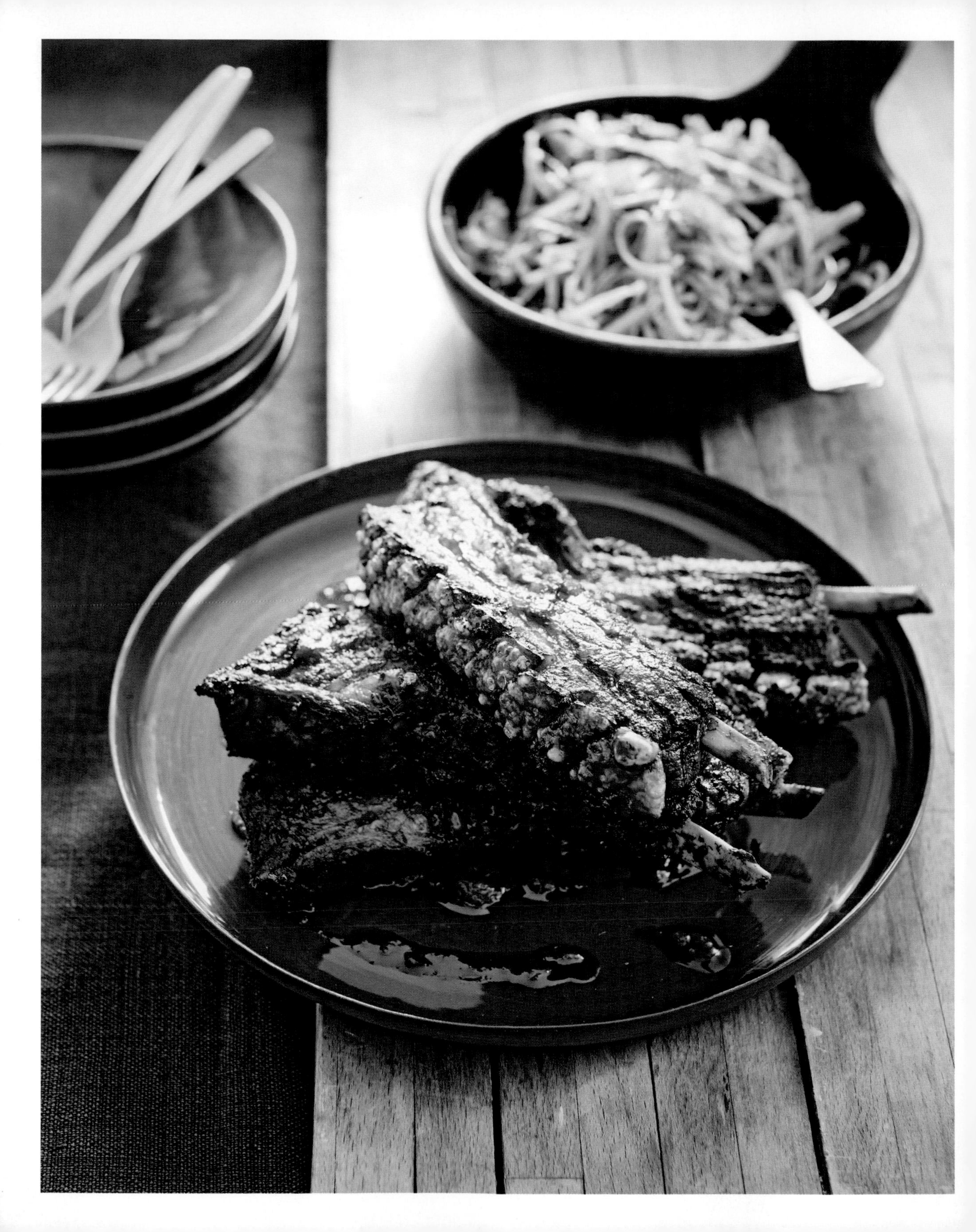

introduction

what is paleo?

The Paleo diet is derived from the foods our ancestors consumed in the Palaeolithic era. It is thought that eating this way suits our genetic make-up better than many of the processed products available in supermarkets today – they are foods we have fuelled our bodies with for centuries that have not been farmed or processed in any way and are therefore absorbed in their raw form. The Paleo shopping list includes: fruits, vegetables, meat, poultry, fish, shellfish, fats, eggs, nuts, seeds, herbs and spices, as well as natural sugars and sweeteners, such as honey. Not on the list are grains (a modern product of agriculture), dairy (processed from animals), refined sugars and blended oils. As a rule of thumb, if you can eat it or buy it in a raw form, you can enjoy it on a Paleo diet.

My approach to Paleo eating is not to tell you the whys or explore the science behind it. I eat Paleo simply because it has made a huge difference to my health and wellbeing. To me, Paleo is about eating nutritionally dense food that is easy to digest and absorb energy from. It's about using good-quality produce and being aware of your body's response to the things you consume. Some people find they have no issue with certain ingredients that are more generally avoided on a Paleo diet – things like oats which are a processed, yet digested easily. The best science when it comes to adapting your diet is to try something and take note of how you feel.

Although there is little evidence of change to our genetic make-up since the Palaeolithic era, there is obvious change in our lifestyle, which I believe makes a drastic difference to what and how we should eat. Our ancestors would have actively hunted and gathered food to fuel their bodies. There would be days of eating very little or nothing at all. And there would be days of complete overindulgence. I think this is something that is commonly misunderstood in modern life. We are told to eat three meals a day, encouraged to eat for many more reasons than simply fuelling our bodies, and food is so readily available that we have little work to do to ensure we are well fed. A simple return to limited, as well as indulgent eating is good for the body.

In Palaeolithic times, on many days our ancestors would have foraged for foods like berries or nuts. On days when hunting went well they would have a whole animal or beehive to gorge on, loading up on mostly proteins but also fats and sugar. This is why it's okay to have days of minimal consumption and days of indulging. There are a variety of dishes in this book designed for clean eating: breakfast bakes, simple salads, as well as slow-roasted main meals. The cakes and treats are high in fat, sugar and protein; a modern version of finding that beehive or that laden nut tree. It does not mean, because it's Paleo, you can eat them every day and I wouldn't advise it. But it does mean that when you do want to indulge you can enjoy something that your body understands, that uses ingredients that won't shock the system. I believe in fasting, I believe in feasting, and I also believe in finding a balance with your diet that suits your lifestyle.

my paleo story

In my eyes, food isn't appreciated enough for its nutritional capabilities. As we learn more about the connection between health and diet, there is no better time to cook and eat Paleo. It's time to take action. I believe in building health through nutrition and instinctively, I have always been into the Paleo way of thinking, I just didn't know that's what it was. When I was a child, I was very fortunate to be brought up on a lot of home-grown produce, I lived with my mum, and our garden was full of fresh fruit and veg. When I stayed with my dad we often visited my grandparents, who were farmers – the joys of hunting down my GarGar and Grandad in their vegetable patch will always be a fond memory. I remember my Grandad for the smell of vine tomatoes and the image of him sat at the kitchen table in his muddy gardening gear, preparing mountains of runner beans to stock the freezer. I enjoyed seeing my food grow, be harvested with care and then to find it on the table in front of me. This is one part of Paleo eating that isn't highlighted enough. I love knowing where my food has come from and I love fresh organic produce – it makes such a difference to the taste of a dish.

As I grew up, I wanted to eat more processed food because that's what everyone had at school: sweets, chocolate and other snacks. When I was 14, I first noticed my body was trying to tell me something. The bloating, pain and discomfort… I remember making a joke of it, calling my tummy 'Mary' my food baby, to make the pain more manageable. But really I was just ignoring the issue. Years of doctor's appointments and research later, I have finally found a system I can work with. I think my body knew from a young age what was good for it, and it decided to tell me.

Now I've given you a little insight to the Paleo way of thinking, but really, in all honesty, it's all just cooking and eating. That is exactly what this book is, it's like any other cookbook but with alternative cooking methods using new and old ingredients. You should consider it a 'normal' way of eating. The second you start to tell yourself you're following a diet and that you're restricted in what you enjoy, you'll make the task of eating well ten times harder for yourself. It's the misunderstanding between dieting and diet.

Food is no longer seen as fuel. Nowadays, we eat because we are hungry, because we are socializing, because we are stressed, bored, tired; we eat to celebrate. Food is a focal point in our lives. Making a change to the way you eat is mentally challenging. See the change as 'normal' and it becomes natural. I know too well how hard dietary changes can be – it doesn't happen overnight. But it does get easier, and I hope that this book helps you along the way. It's definitely been a huge stepping-stone in my dietary progression and I have learnt a lot.

I want this book to encourage and motivate people with specific dietary requirements; but I also want it to be helpful to those who may have to cater for the dietary needs of others, showing that food doesn't have to be restrictive and that you can still sit down and have a three-course meal with a side of Paleo bread and a chocolate dessert at the end.

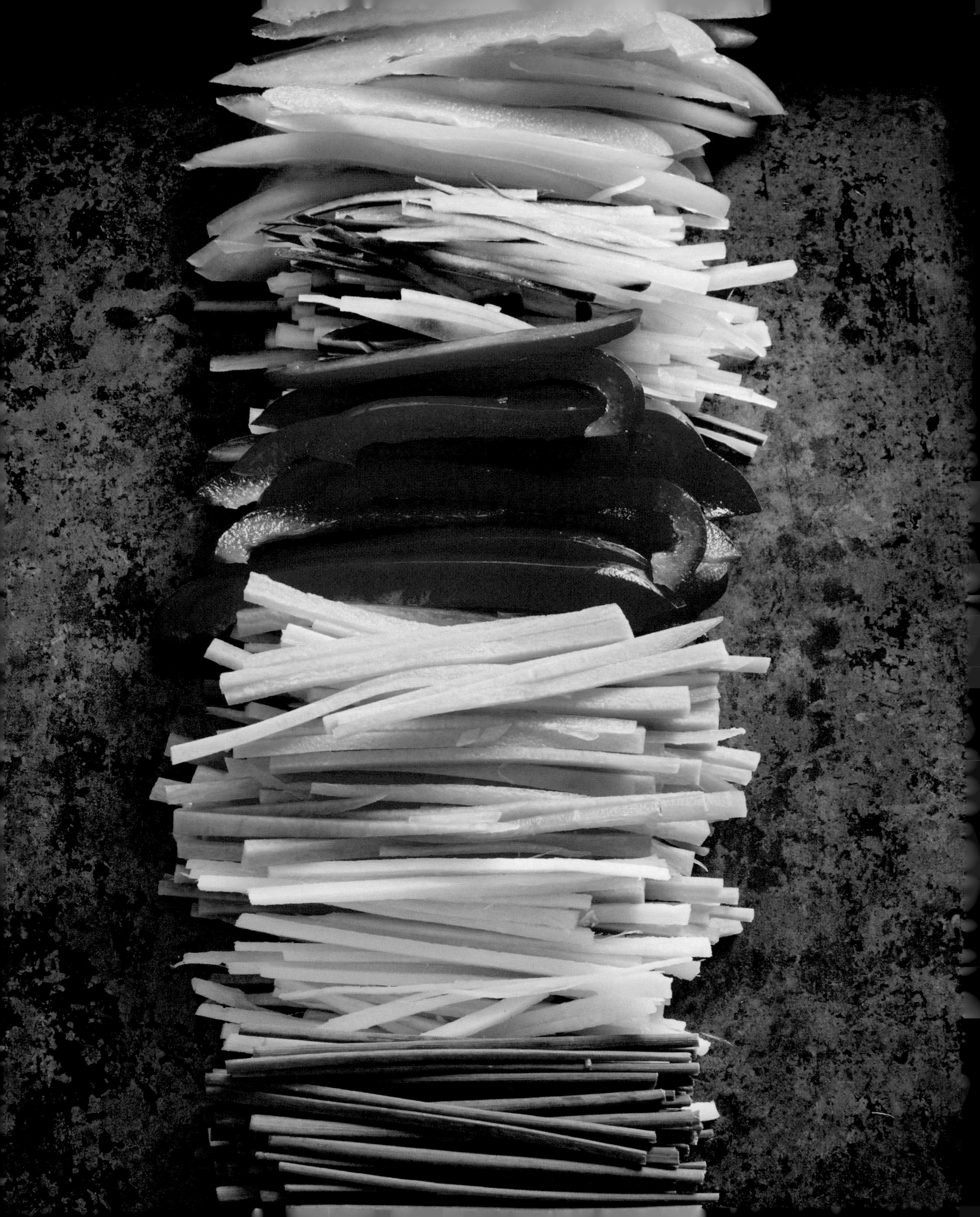

top 10 tips

Rehydrate each morning

Mix the juice of ½ lemon into a glass of water and drink it when you wake up. This gets your digestive system ready for the day ahead. It might seem obvious but digestion is so important when it comes to your diet – if you aren't digesting the food you eat properly, you aren't absorbing its nutrients either. Throughout the day, drink more water, more than you might think, and up the herbal teas and fresh vegetable juices.

Cook with solid fats

Solid fats are easily identifiable because they are solid at room temperature, for example; coconut oil, duck fat, beef dripping and pork fat (or lard). They are great for cooking with as they don't get damaged by heat and can add flavour.

Be adventurous

The more adventurous you are with seasonings, ingredients and cooking techniques, the more exciting and fulfilling your food will be. Don't be afraid to experiment with your cooking.

Try the Paleo 4:2:1

Eat mostly vegetables and protein (eggs, fish and shellfish as these are easier for the gut to break down than other meats and poultry) for four days in a week, mostly vegetables for two days in a week, leaving one day in the week to indulge. I developed this weekly ratio while writing this book, when I was constantly taste-testing the recipes to make sure they were just right and eating all types of foods in one day – foods that were nutritious but sometimes I would test recipes all day that were high in sugar or fat, and my body really didn't like it (remember, it's about striking a balance!). You can alter the order of these days in any way you like, change it weekly, but ensure that the ratio is right for you. Be aware on days when you are indulging that nuts are often a replacement for flour and can sometimes be difficult to digest.

Don't give up

If you make a change and it doesn't give you the results you want straight away, persevere and try again or try something different. Everybody is different and every body is different, but food can be a remedy for many things. Allow time for a new routine to show results and for your body to adjust to any changes you are making.

Leave plenty of time between meals

This allows your body enough time to digest and absorb the food you consume. It's very important to make time to enjoy your meals, chew slowly and properly. Try not to drink while you eat as it dilutes your digestive enzymes and stomach acids that aid the digestion process.

Keep things balanced

Limit the amount of fat, sugar, carbohydrate and protein you eat throughout the day. Think about what the right balance is for you when planning meals.

Cook at home as much as possible

This is the only way to know exactly what is in your food and allows you to make full use of the produce you buy. For example, make stock and bone broth using the bones from a roast chicken – it is a great way to use every part of the bird and limits the temptation to use processed stocks in soups and sauces.

Take small steps to change your diet

Find one thing at a time that works for you and steadily introduce new ingredients – it can be as simple as trying nut, hemp or coconut milk instead of dairy; or not using white refined sugar but a natural alternative like honey. Small steps make change manageable.

Invest in a good-quality non-stick pan

This is such a great invention and means you don't always have to add fats to prepare your food.

ingredients

Meat, fish and poultry

Meat is a real staple food in Paleo eating, in fact I know many people who eat just protein and veg and they don't fuss with much else. It's always best to go for organic, free-range, grass-fed and local, as the nutritional value is much greater. You want to consume the best quality meat for both health and flavour. The same rules apply for fish, however try to buy wild line-caught fish. It's no secret that many fishing methods have been destructive of our oceans, so source your ingredients responsibly.

Eggs

Eggs are a great source of protein, omega-3 fatty acids, as well as vitamins and minerals. They should be included in a balanced diet, especially for vegetarian Paleo eaters. As with meat, it's important to buy fresh, organic, free-range eggs for the nutritional benefits. Like everything else on the Paleo diet, consume eggs in moderation to avoid developing intolerances.

Fruit and vegetables

Vegetables are my favourite food group and I think they are often underestimated. From an array of colours, I know my plate will be packed full of goodness and loaded with different vitamins and minerals that are found in the presence of colour. Everyone that assumes I follow a low- or no-carb diet because I don't consume grains asks, 'where do I get my energy from?' The answer, 'fruit and vegetables!' In the most basic of terms, you get a sugar buzz from fruit (a fast carb) and quick boost of energy, and vegetables (slower carbs) release energy over a longer period of time. There are different nutritional values to each vegetable, for instance sweet potatoes are a high-carb substance, so be aware of the make-up of different ingredients. As ever, buy fresh, organic, seasonal and local produce for the best quality.

Nuts and seeds

Loaded with healthy fats, vitamins and minerals, nuts and seeds are a great addition to the Paleo plate. They are great in bakes, as a snack or with breakfast, just keep in mind that they do not need to be consumed daily or with every meal. Nuts and seeds should be consumed in moderation because they can be quite hard to digest and can make it difficult for the body to absorb nutrients from other ingredients.

Solid fats

Low-fat diets are over. We should embrace fats and encourage consumption of good-quality fats. Use solid fats (ones that are solid at room temperature) like unrefined coconut oil, lard, beef dripping, duck fat, and goose fat for cooking and heating. Use avocado, olive, nut and sesame oils for dressing dishes and adding flavour. I believe that when I first included more fats in my diet, my hair grew thicker and longer.

Natural sugars

Sugar is my hardest battle; natural sugars such as honey, fruit syrups, maple syrup and palm sugar are great replacements for refined white sugar. However, I don't believe they add much nutritional value to my plate. They are great for fulfilling a sugar craving and for giving you a quick burst of energy, but ultimately they are good for my wellbeing because I have a sweet tooth and enjoy my treats. Don't be afraid to indulge in the things you enjoy from time to time.

Ingredients to avoid

The Paleo diet does not allow the consumption of any grains, including wheat, barley, freekeh and so on. Legumes (beans, including soy products, and podded peas) should also be avoided. Dairy and soy products should be replaced with nut and seed milks and cheeses, while refined sugars and processed oils, including sunflower and vegetable oils, should be avoided altogether. These ingredients can be inflammatory and so can lead to poor gut health. Some people choose to include sprouted grains, such as sprouted wild rice in their diet, but tread carfeully whenever you make a dietary change. Some people also find they can include oats or corn, or other 'no-go' ingredients in their diet without adverse effects, so see what works for you and go from there.

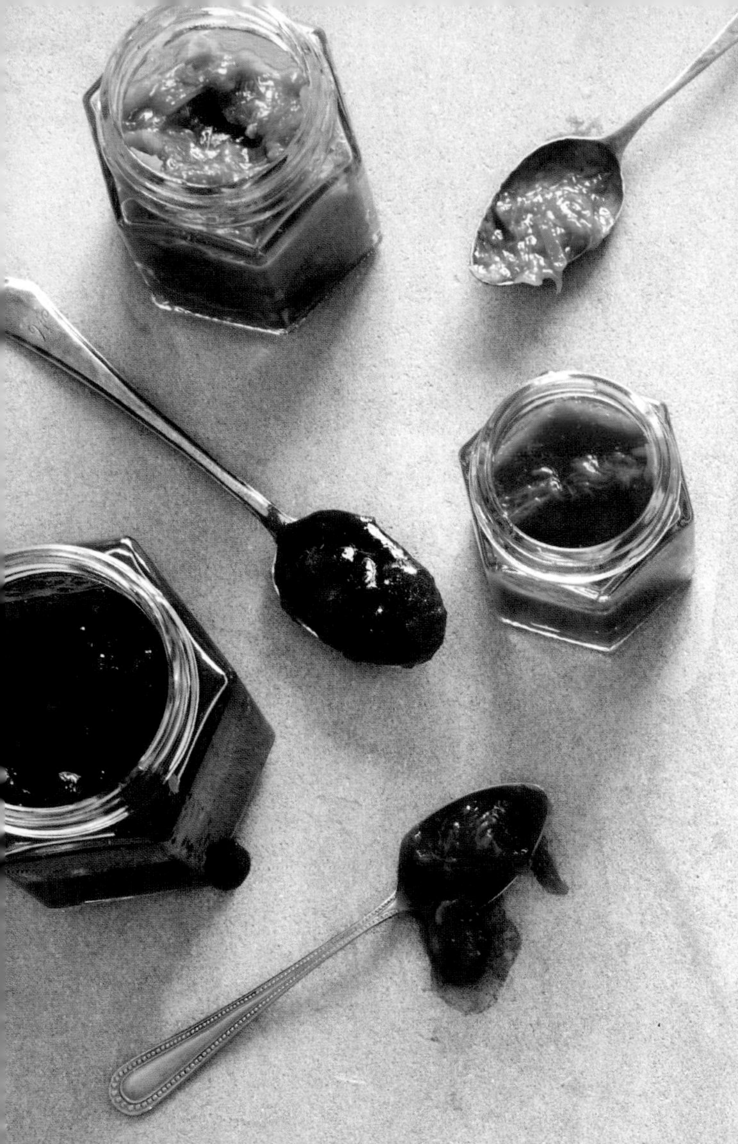

marmalade

10 large oranges
honey (or your choice of Paleo sweetener), to taste
a 320-g/11-oz. capacity sterilized glass jar with airtight lid

MAKES 1 JAR

With a small, sharp knife peel the skin of 2–4 of the oranges, depending on how much peel you like in the preserve. Remove the pith and thinly slice the peel.

Top and tail the remaining oranges and remove the skin, including the white pith. Cut into segments and put the segments, peel and generous squeeze of sweetener into a saucepan but keep all the off-cuts and pips. Squeeze the excess juice from the off-cuts into the pan and set over medium heat.

Bring the mixture to a simmer until it turns thick and sticky. You may need to add a little water to avoid it sticking to the pan. As it simmers the excess water steams off, however you don't want to dilute your oranges too much so only add a little at a time if you must. You may also need to taste test for sweetness as you go along, adding 5–10 tablespoons of sweetener as desired – take care, the mixture will be very hot.

Transfer to the sterilized glass jar, screw on the lid and turn upside-down while warm – the pressure created while cooling will seal the jar. Store in the fridge.

preserves

My Paleo preserves are a lot like compotes. Fruits with a higher sugar content naturally last longer in the fridge than others and the pectin content in fruits with stones/pits and seeds helps them to set.

summer berry

800 g/1¾ lbs. mixed fresh or frozen strawberries, blueberries and raspberries, strawberries halved

natural sweetener, such as fresh apple juice, honey or pure maple syrup (optional)

2 x 227-g/8-oz. capacity sterilized glass jars with airtight lids

MAKES 2 JARS

Put the mixed berries into a saucepan and add 50 ml/3½ tablespoons of water. The water helps the fruit not to stick to the pan before it starts to produce liquid. Bring to a simmer over a medium heat. When the fruit has cooked down a bit and has produced quite a bit of liquid turn up the heat to a constant but gentle boil for about 10 minutes. Stir occasionally to ensure the fruit is distributed evenly and doesn't stick to the pan. Turn back down to a simmer for 5–10 minutes – you will notice the bubbles slow as the mixture thickens.

Taste test for sweetness, add sweetener as desired but take care, the mixture will be very hot. Drop a teaspoon of the mixture onto a cold plate, then run a spoon through the middle of the mixture and, if ready, it should leave a canal. Pour into sterilized jars, seal and store following the instruction for Marmalade (left).

plum and cinnamon

400 g/14 oz. plums

1 cinnamon stick

honey (or your choice of Paleo sweetener), to taste

a 227-g/8-oz. capacity sterilized glass jar with airtight lid

MAKES 1 JAR

Start by cutting the plums in half and removing the stone/pit. Set the stones/pits aside and put the plums in a saucepan with enough water to come halfway up.

Add the cinnamon and a squeeze or two of honey depending on how sweet you want the jam/jelly and set over medium heat. I always include the stones/pits here as it helps to set the mixture. Bring to a gentle simmer, until the fruit starts to break down.

Remove the pan from the heat and leave to cool, for the flavours to infuse and the jam to set slightly. Pass through a fine-mesh sieve/strainer, using the back of a spoon to press the mixture through and release more juices. Discard the stones/pits and cinnamon stick. Return any remaining fruit pulp left in the sieve/strainer to the mixture.

Pour into sterilized jars, seal following the instruction for Marmalade (left) and store in the fridge.

gooseberry

250 g/9 oz. fresh or frozen gooseberries

a squeeze of fresh lemon juice

50 g/2½ tablespoons strawberry sugar-free preserve (I use St. Dalfour)

honey (or your choice of Paleo sweetener), to taste

a 227-g/8-oz. capacity sterilized glass jar with airtight lid

MAKES 1 JAR

Heat all the ingredients in a saucepan set over medium heat for roughly 20 minutes, give or take, keeping an eye on the mixture and stirring occasionally – you don't want the mix to become too thick!

Test and seal following the instruction for Marmalade (left) and store in the fridge.

apple and rhubarb

3 apples

a 1-cm/⅜-inch piece of fresh ginger

350 g/12 oz. fresh rhubarb, sliced

honey (or your choice of Paleo sweetener), to taste

a 227-g/8-oz. capacity sterilized glass jar with airtight lid

MAKES 1 JAR

Start by coring the apples. Wrap and tie the cores in muslin/cheesecloth and set aside. Juice the remaining apple flesh with the some ginger – you need 200 g/¾ cup juice – and pour into a saucepan.

Add the sliced rhubarb and wrapped apple cores, and bring to a boil over medium heat until the liquid evaporates slightly and the mixture thickens. The bubbles will slow as an indication that it is almost ready. Carefully taste the mixture halfway through the cooking process (allow it to cool on a spoon before doing so) to see if and how much honey to add.

Pour into sterilized jars, seal following the instruction for Marmalade (left) and store in the fridge.

sauces and sides

herbed mayo

2 egg yolks

$^{1}/_{2}$–1 lemon

1 tablespoon white wine (or cider) vinegar

$^{1}/_{2}$ teaspoon Dijon (or English) mustard

240 ml/1 cup light olive oil

120 ml/$^{1}/_{2}$ cup extra virgin olive oil

a handful of chopped fresh dill

a handful of chopped fresh parsley

1 spring onion/scallion, thinly sliced (optional)

salt and black pepper, to season

MAKES 360 ML/1 $^{1}/_{2}$ CUPS

Put the egg yolk in a narrow container with high sides (a measuring jug/pitcher is ideal) with a squeeze of lemon, the vinegar, mustard and a little salt and pepper. Whiz together using a handheld electric blender, then slowly pour in the oils a little at a time. I pour a little then blend, pour a little then blend, and continue until I have the right consistency. Stir in the chopped herbs and spring onion/scallion (if using), season to taste and serve.

Alternatively use good-quality free range mayonnaise, add herbs, season to taste and serve.

honey butter

Paleo butter (I use coconut butter or Biona Organic Cocomega coconut spread)

honey, to taste

Spoon the required amount of Paleo butter into a small mixing bowl and bring to room temperature.

When softened, add a little honey and mix well. Taste and add a little more honey if desired.

Spread on warm toast or fruit buns (page 50).

garlic mayo

1 egg yolk

$^{1}/_{2}$ lemon

1 teaspoon white wine (or cider) vinegar

$^{1}/_{2}$ teaspoon Dijon (or English) mustard

120 ml/$^{1}/_{2}$ cup light olive oil

60 ml/$^{1}/_{4}$ cup extra virgin olive oil

1–2 garlic cloves, crushed

salt and black pepper, to season

MAKES 180 ML/ $^{3}/_{4}$ CUP

Put the egg yolk in a narrow container with high sides (a measuring jug/pitcher is ideal) with a squeeze of lemon, the vinegar, mustard and a little salt and pepper. Whiz together using a handheld electric blender, then slowly pour in the oils a little at a time. I pour a little then blend, pour a little then blend, and continue until I have the right consistency. Stir in the crushed garlic and serve.

Alternatively use good-quality free range mayonnaise and add the garlic, season to taste and serve.

apple sauce

350 g/3$^{1}/_{2}$ cups cored and chopped apples

freshly squeezed juice of $^{1}/_{2}$ lemon

600 ml/2$^{1}/_{2}$ cups pure apple juice

1–2 star anise

MAKES 250 ML/1 CUP

Put all of the ingredients in a saucepan and set over medium heat. Bring to a simmer and cook until the apple pieces break down and the lemon and apple juice reduces by a third.

Remove the pan from the heat. Cool and store in the fridge until ready to serve.

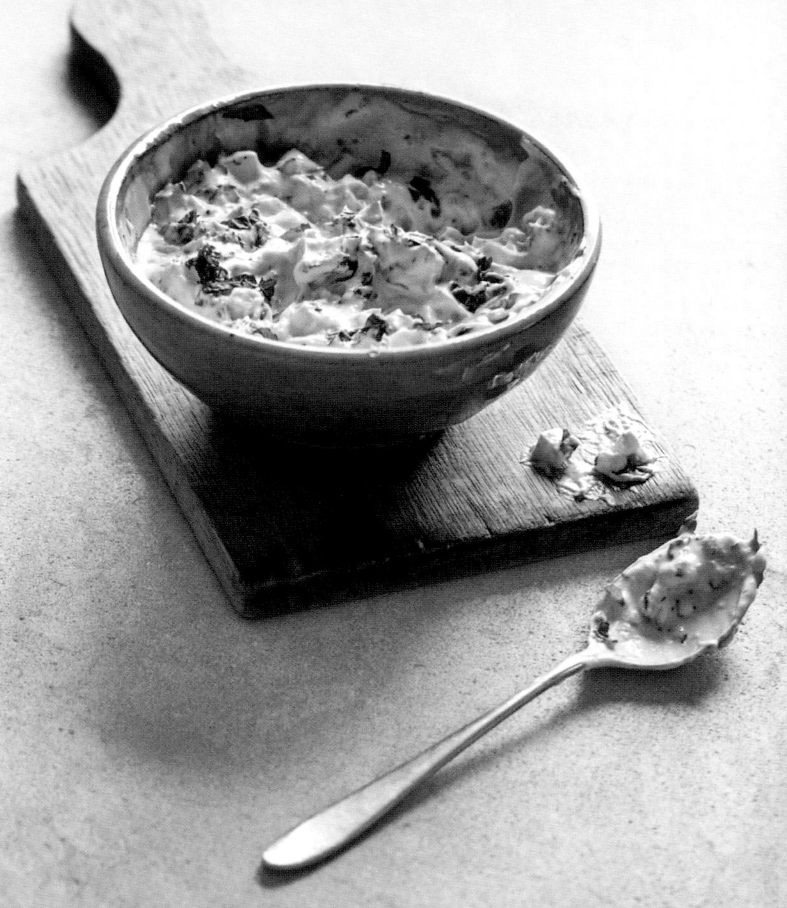

tzatziki

the solidified coconut from a can of coconut milk or cream (see Note)

1–2 garlic cloves, crushed

1/3 cucumber, deseeded and finely diced

a small handful of fresh mint leaves, finely chopped

grated zest and freshly squeezed juice of 1 lemon

salt and black pepper, to season

SERVES 2–4

Using a can of coconut milk from the fridge (so that the creamy part has risen to the top and solidified) for the tzatziki gives a lovely creamy consistency (see Note). Put the solidified cream in a mixing bowl and whip it to the consistency of lightly whipped cream.

Add the remaining ingredients (I would advise starting with 1 garlic clove) and mix well.

Taste the tzatziki – the lemon zest and juice should cut through the heavy coconut flavour, so add more if not. Season to taste and set aside until ready to serve.

Note: To split the coconut milk or cream in the can, put the unopened can in the fridge for an hour or two, or even overnight. When you open it, the cream will have come to the top of the can and the water will be at the bottom. Drain the liquid and use the cream as instructed in the method.

mustard slaw

1 kohlrabi (or turnip), grated or very thinly sliced

1 head of broccoli, grated or very thinly sliced

1 carrot, grated or very thinly sliced

1 celery stalk/rib, thinly sliced

1/4 red or white cabbage, grated or very thinly sliced

freshly squeezed juice of 1/2 lemon

olive oil, to drizzle

1–2 teaspoons wholegrain mustard, to taste

SERVES 2–4

Put all of the grated or sliced vegetables in a large mixing bowl and squeeze over the lemon juice. Mix well then drizzle with olive oil and stir in a little mustard. Taste, adding more mustard if you like, season with salt and pepper and set aside. For a creamier slaw use mayonnaise instead of oil.

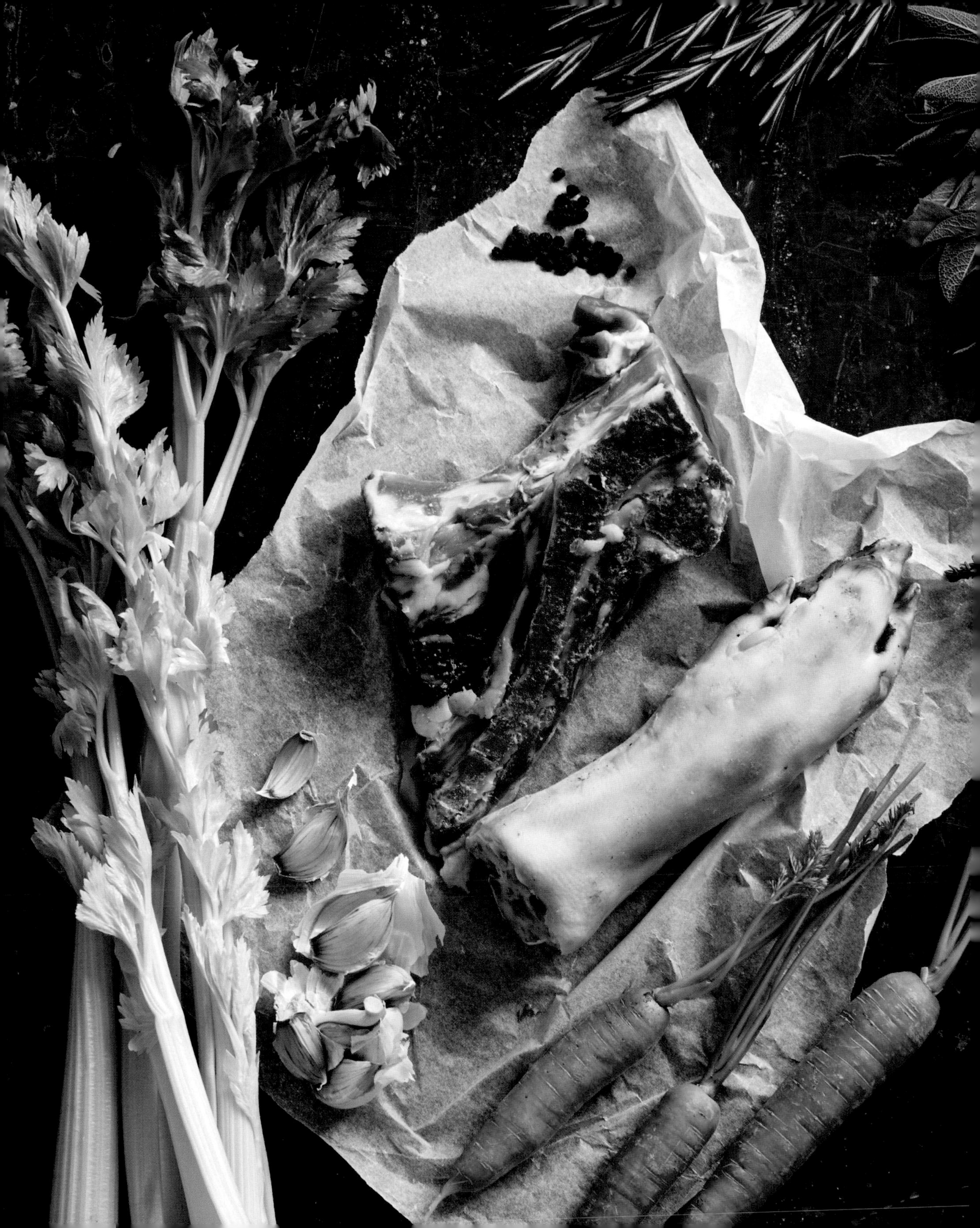

bone broth

Bone broth has endless amounts of benefits. It's full of collagen, glutamine, calcium, magnesium and glucosamine, making it amazing for your gut, skin, joints, immune system and metabolism. Ask your butcher to cut the bone so all the nutrients inside it are released more easily.

1 pig's foot
1 pork bone
1 carrot
2 celery stalks/ribs
1 onion, cut in half
a few sprigs of fresh sage, rosemary and thyme
1 teaspoon black peppercorns
1 garlic clove

MAKES ABOUT 500 ML/
2 CUPS

Put all the ingredients in a large saucepan, cover with water and a lid and bring to a boil over medium heat. Lower the heat and simmer for 1–2 hours. Skim the top of any excess foam.

For best results you should transfer this liquid and the ingredients to a container, cool, seal and set in the fridge overnight, then bring to the boil again the next day, but you could skip this part.

You can do this a day or two before using as you can store it in the fridge until you are ready to use it, for up to 3 days and the freezer for up to 1 month.

Use the broth as a base for soups by adding any ingredients you would like to produce a hearty and rejuvenating broth.

vegetable stock

Vegetable stock is great to use in sauces, soups, for poaching, or even boiling to add extra flavour to dishes. And it's super-easy to make so there's no reason to buy bouillon cubes that are often laden with nasty preservatives.

2 medium carrots
1/2 white onion (skin on)
2 bay leaves
2 sprigs of fresh rosemary
1 tablespoon black peppercorns
5 sprigs of fresh thyme
2 celery stalks/ribs
1/2 leek
a broccoli stalk (optional)
2 garlic cloves (skin on)

MAKES ABOUT 500 ML/
2 CUPS

Trim and chop all the ingredients so that they fit in a medium–large saucepan.

Set the pan with vegetables over medium heat and pour over enough water to cover everything. Simmer for a minimum of 2 hours or longer if you want a stronger tasting stock. Strain through a fine-mesh sieve/strainer into a jug/pitcher or airtight container if storing to use another time.

Use right away or store in the fridge for up to 3 days and the freezer for up to 1 month.

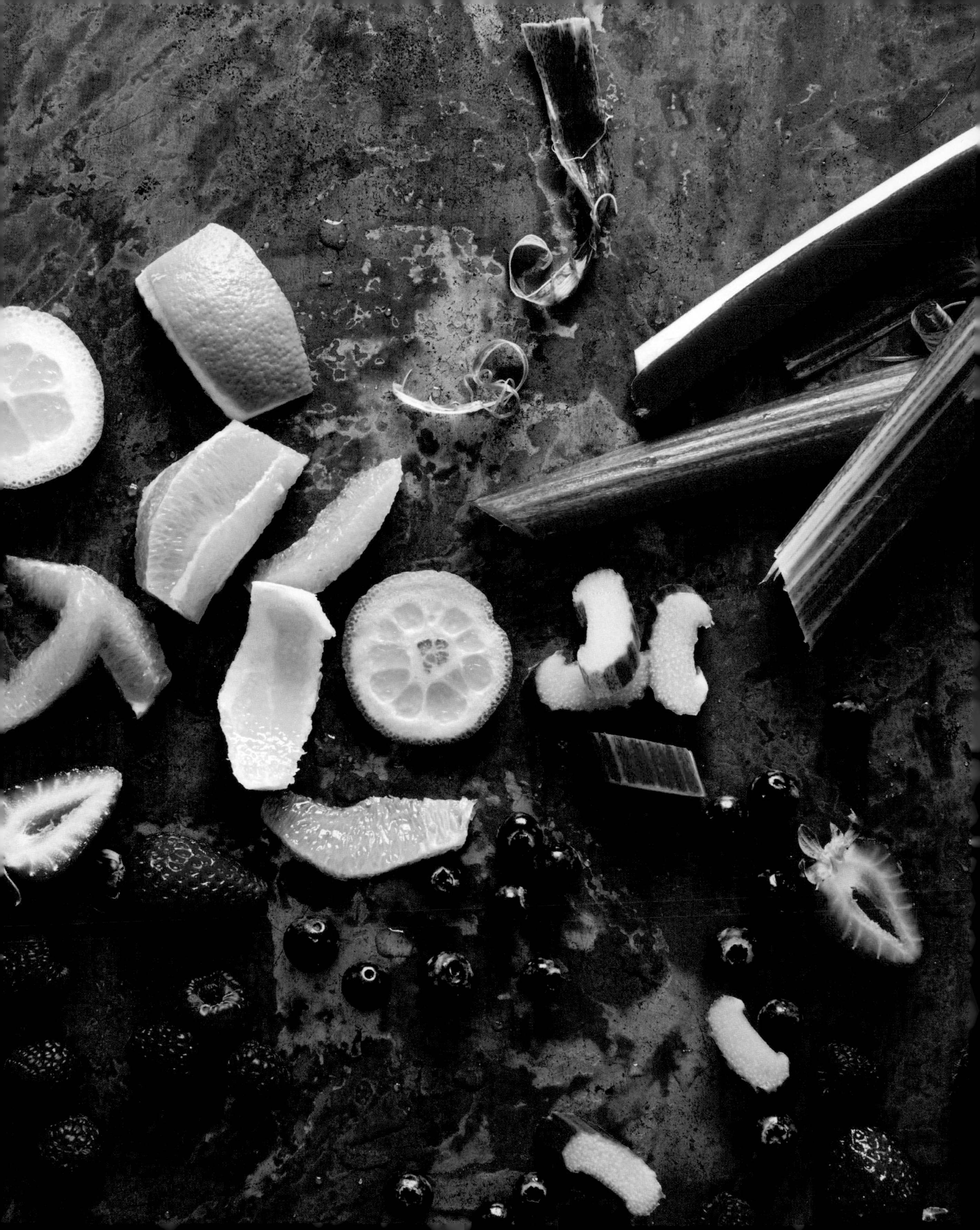

breakfast boost

We are often told that breakfast is the most important meal of the day. When I first started eating Paleo it was the meal I grew bored of the quickest; I always just relied on an egg with a bit of spinach and bacon. I hope this chapter inspires you and offers plenty of options so that breakfast can still be versatile.

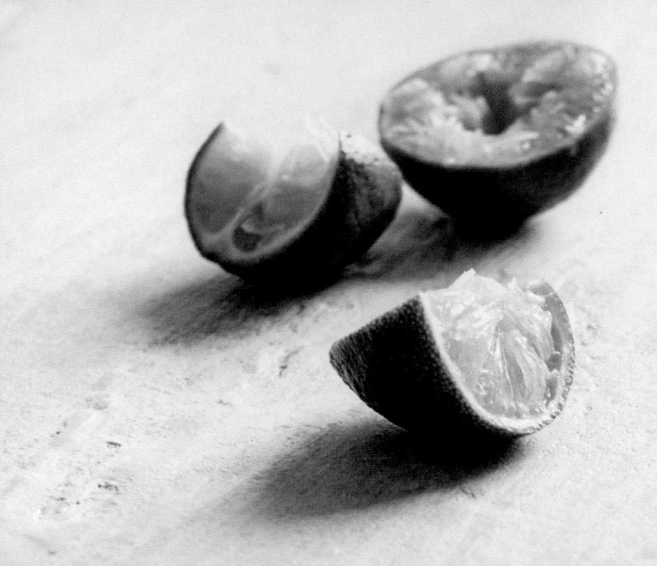

breakfast smoothies

I love a smoothie. If the colours go together the flavours normally do, too! These are two of my more fruity favourites. Try to limit the fruit in smoothies as it's easy to get carried away and just make them a sugar fix. Instead focus on nutrient-rich vegetables for a healthy start to the day.

pretty and pink

a handful of fresh or frozen raspberries
1/2 apple (or a dash of fresh apple juice, to taste)
1 carrot
a big squeeze of lemon
a 2.5-cm/1-inch piece of ginger
a wedge of fresh beetroot/beet
1/2 avocado (optional)

a high-powered blender (I use a NutriBullet)

MAKES 1

Add all the ingredients to the high-powered blender. Cover with water and blitz to combine.

The avocado is optional – without it the smoothie can be a bit too fibrous. Alternatively you can strain it to make a breakfast juice – blitz with ice at the end to make it slushy!

go green

150 ml/2/3 cup coconut milk
a large handful of fresh spinach
juice of 1/2 lime
1 pineapple slice
1/2–1 banana, depending on size

a high-powered blender (I use a NutriBullet)

MAKES 1

Add all the ingredients to the high-powered blender. The longer you leave it the smoother the consistency.

Add a drop of water for more juice-like consistency and for extra hydration of course! Best served with ice.

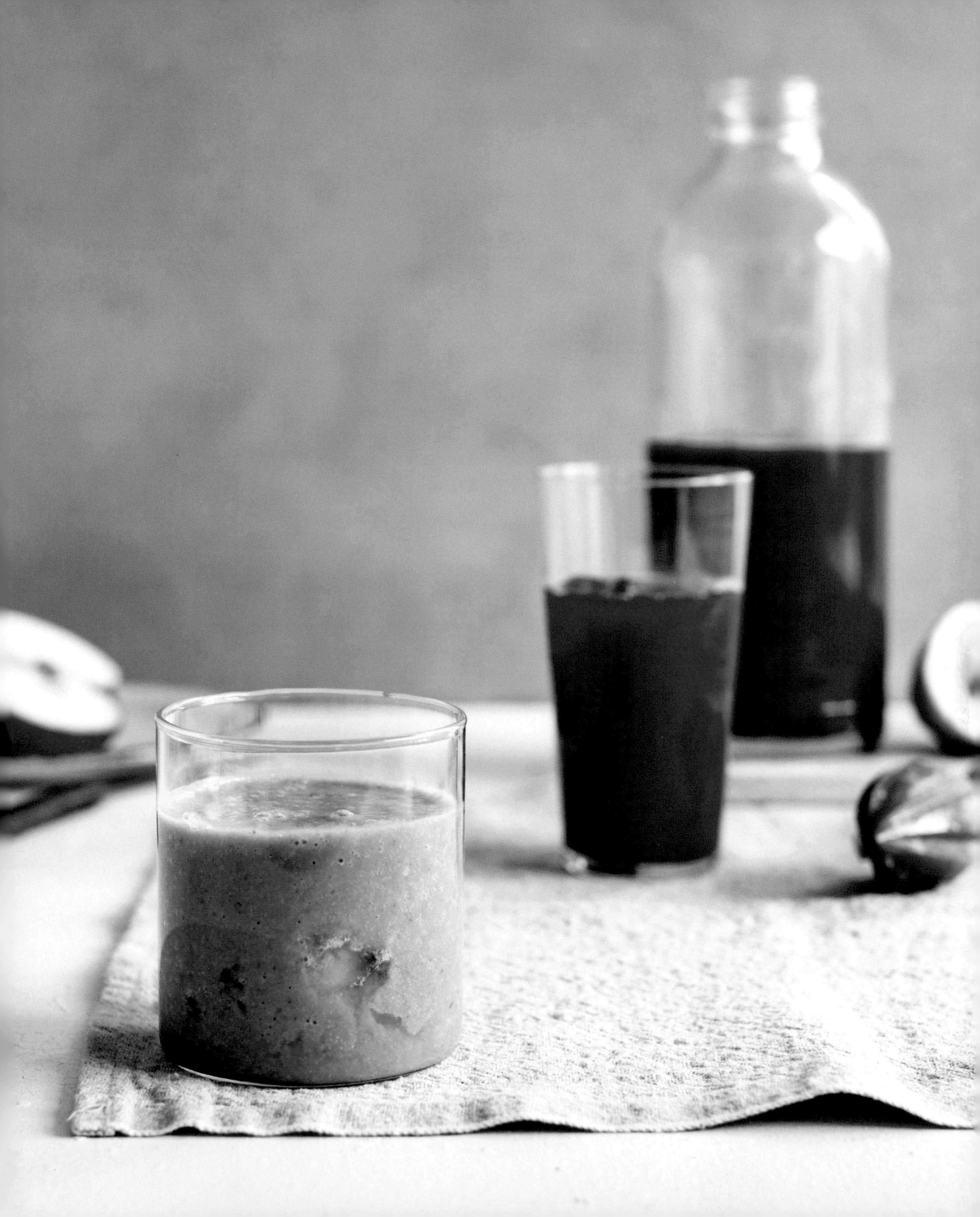

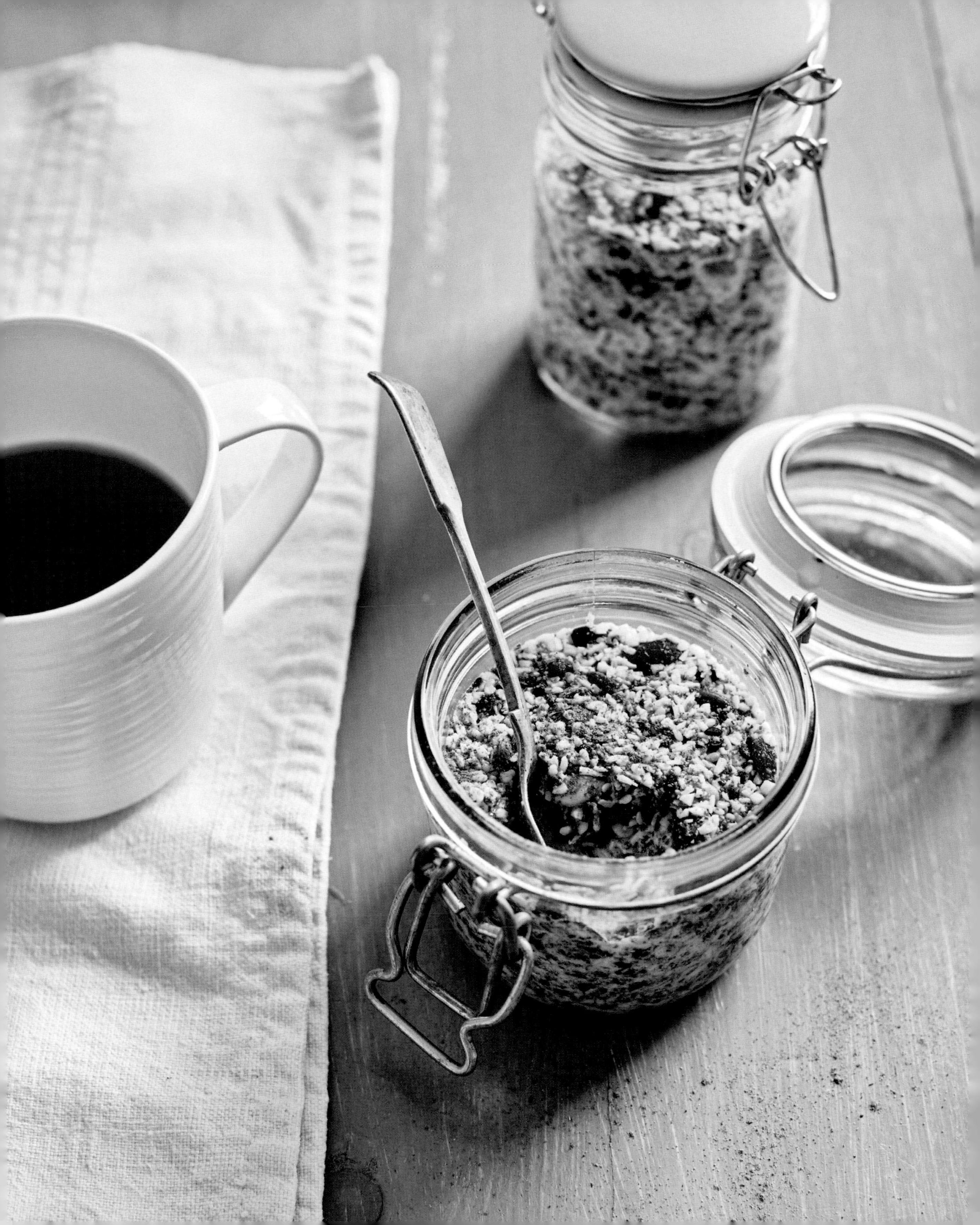

overnight seed pots

I love an overnight pot – it means breakfast is ready on busy days. In writing this book I've found it extremely handy having a friend as my own personal nutritional tutor and learnt that soaking nuts and seeds helps to de-activate enzyme inhibitors. These substances are naturally present in nuts and seeds, which protect them from digestion in the stomach. Thank you, Holly!

mixed seed pot

10 g/1 heaped tablespoon milled flaxseeds/ linseeds

10 g/1 heaped tablespoon mixed sesame seeds

15 g/1 1/2 tablespoons mixed sunflower and pumpkin seeds

10 g/1 tablespoon desiccated/shredded coconut

5 g/1 tablespoon goji berries

70 ml/1/3 cup hemp milk (or other Paleo milk of choice, see page 11)

SERVES 1

Mix all the ingredients together in a container with a lid, cover and leave in the fridge overnight.

By morning, the seeds, coconut and berries will have plumped up with hemp milk and can be enjoyed at home or on the go.

Note: You can double, triple or quadruple the quantities of ingredients here if you want to prepare more than one serving. The mixture will keep for up to 3 days in the fridge.

chia pot

15 g/1 tablespoon chia seeds

85 g/1/3 cup almond milk (or other Paleo milk of choice, see page 11)

seeds from 1 vanilla pod/bean

1 tablespoon almond butter

flaked/slivered almonds, to serve

SERVES 1

Mix all the ingredients together in a container with a lid, stir a few times in the first 30 minutes. Leave in the fridge and enjoy in the morning.

Add some flaked/slivered almonds for added texture and serve.

Note: You can double, triple or quadruple the quantities of ingredients here if you want to prepare more than one serving. The mixture will keep for up to 3 days in the fridge.

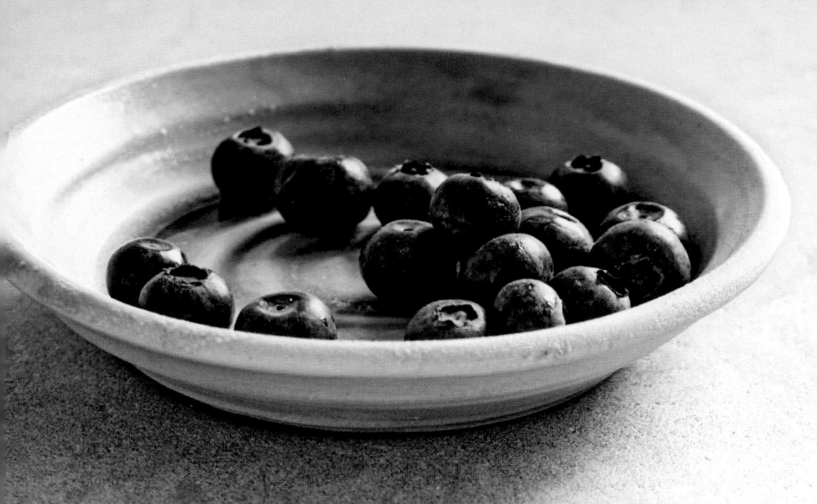

banana and blueberry seed muffins

The batter for this recipe makes enough for 12 muffins or 16 cupcakes. If making them cupcake-size, I like to make 12 at a time (one pan worth) and refrigerate the rest of the batter to turn into pancakes the next day. Serve them warm from the oven.

100 g/$^{3}/_{4}$ cup flaxseeds/ linseeds

130 g/1$^{1}/_{3}$ cups ground almonds

50 g/$^{1}/_{2}$ cup almond flour

40 g/$^{1}/_{3}$ cup tapioca flour

30 g/$^{1}/_{4}$ cup poppy seeds

1$^{1}/_{2}$ teaspoons bicarbonate of/baking soda

60 g/$^{1}/_{4}$ cup pure maple syrup

20 g/1 tablespoon date syrup

2 eggs

1 teaspoon vanilla extract

60 g/$^{1}/_{3}$ cup almond oil

200 g/$^{3}/_{4}$ cup unsweetened almond milk

130 g/$^{2}/_{3}$ cup mashed banana

40 g/$^{1}/_{3}$ cup fresh blueberries

salt, to season

a 12-hole muffin pan lined with paper cases

MAKES 12

Preheat the oven to 170°C (325°F) Gas 3.

Start by blitzing the flaxseeds and ground almonds together – I use my NutriBullet for this but you could use a pestle and mortar or food processor. It should transform into something like wholemeal/whole-wheat flour.

Mix together all the dry ingredients including the ground flaxseeds and almonds in a large mixing bowl.

In a separate mixing bowl, whisk the syrups and eggs together until they start to lighten up (if you don't have date syrup in the cupboard just use 80 g/ 4 tablespoons maple syrup). Add the vanilla, almond oil and milk, and whisk again. Then add the mashed banana.

Make a well in the dry ingredients and pour in the eggy mixture, add a pinch of salt and bring everything together using a handheld electric whisk. Once the ingredients are well combined, stir in the blueberries.

Fill each muffin case and bake in the preheated oven for 15–20 minutes.

Remove from the oven and cool the muffins on a wire rack. Serve.

Note: If you are reserving some of the batter for pancakes the next day, store it in the fridge but bring to room temperature before frying as you would the banana pancakes on page 31.

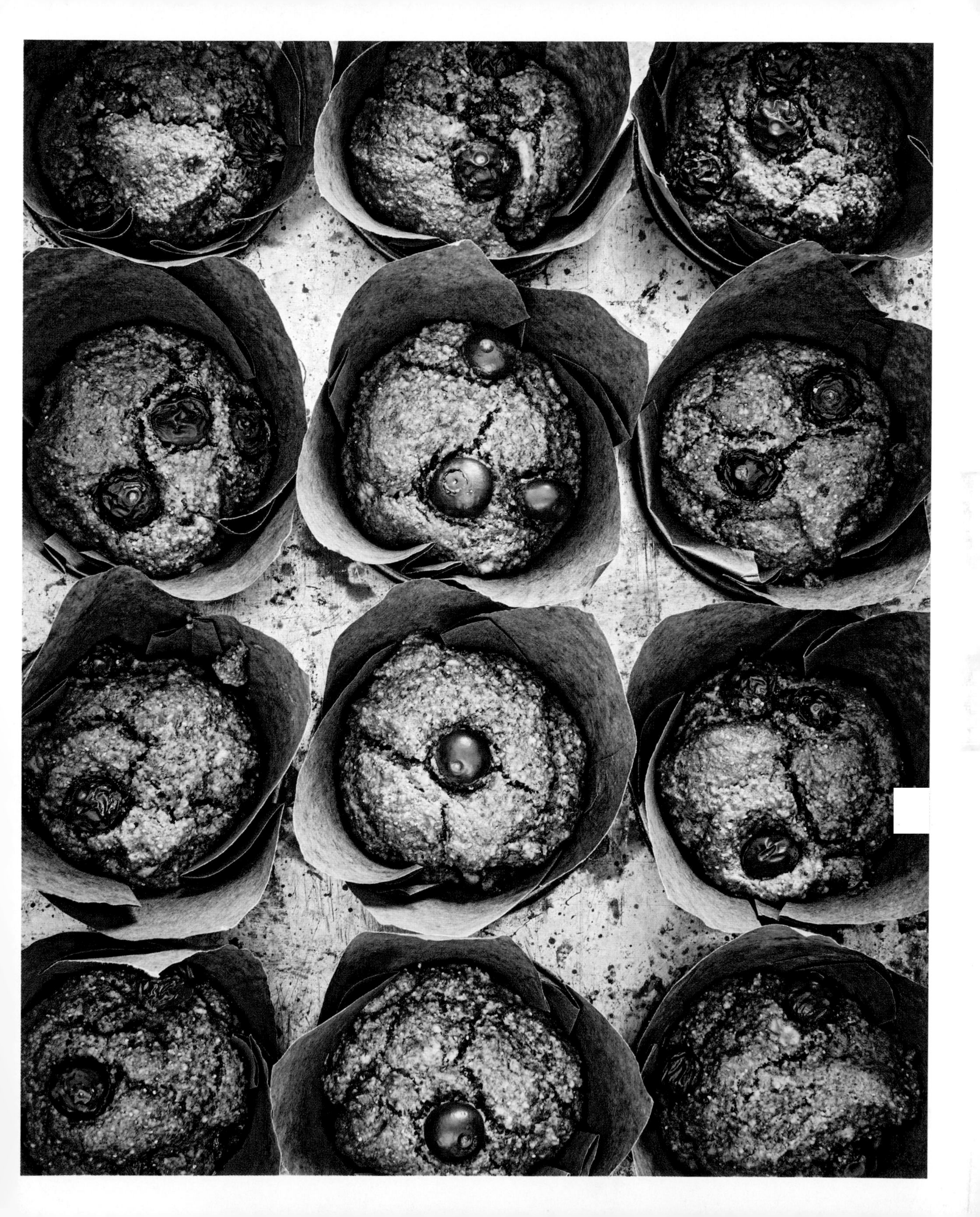

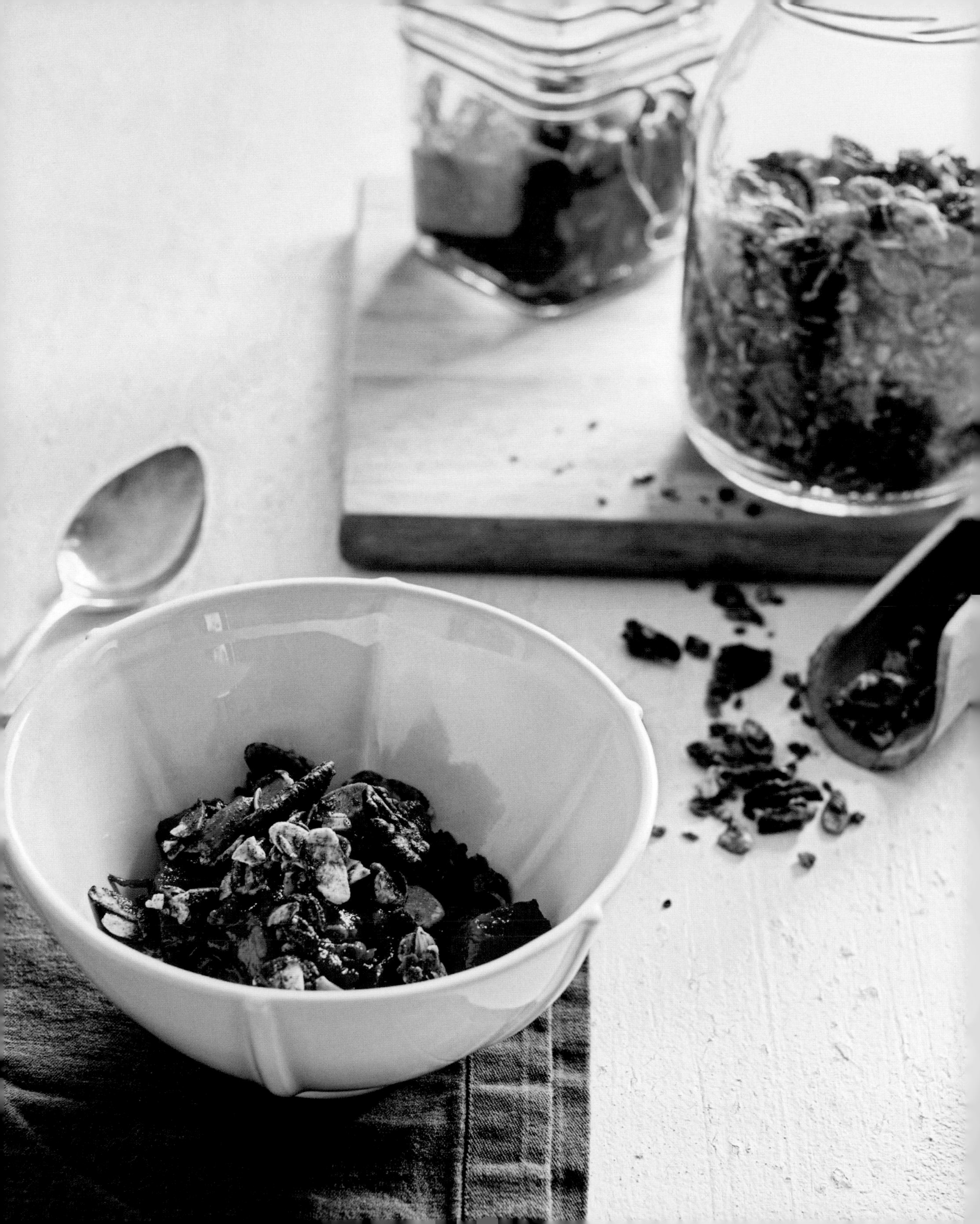

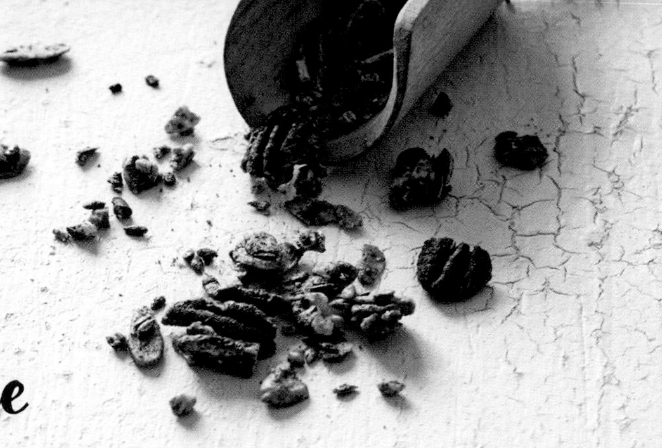

cinnamon 'granola' with pear and cranberry compote

You'd be forgiven for thinking granola would be out on a Paleo diet but this grain-free recipe is a great cereal option, served hot or cold. I like to make the compote in large batches and store it in the freezer ready to defrost and serve in no time. It's also great as a pudding, just heat the fruit, add a little custard (page 112) and you are good to go.

200 g/1 1/2 cups pecans, roughly chopped

100 g/1 1/4 cups flaked/slivered almonds

60 g/1/2 cup mixed chopped nuts

50 g/1/3 cup brown flaxseeds/linseeds

2–3 tablespoons pure maple syrup

2–3 teaspoons ground cinnamon

pear and cranberry compote

8 pears, cored and roughly chopped

grated zest and freshly squeezed juice of 1 lemon

2–4 tablespoons pure maple syrup (optional)

80 g/3/4 cup fresh or dried cranberries

sterilized glass jars with airtight lids (optional)

a baking sheet lined with baking parchment

SERVES 4

First make the compote. Put the chopped pears, lemon zest and juice into a saucepan. Set over medium heat and simmer for 10–15 minutes, until the fruit becomes soft and breaks up easily when pressed with the back of a spoon. You may need to add a little water depending how ripe your pears are, or add a little maple syrup if you have a sweet tooth. The cooking time and the amount of water all depends on how ripe your pears are and how well you like them cooked. Some days I like them to reach a mash consistency, others I like to keep whole bits of pears.

If using fresh cranberries, put 2 tablespoons of maple syrup with 200 ml/¾ cup of water in a separate pan, add the cranberries and set over medium heat. Cook for 10–15 minutes until the berries break down, and produce a luscious red syrup. Carefully taste the syrup (let a little cool on a spoon first) and add more maple syrup if desired. Set aside.

Mix the pear mixture into the cranberry mixture (or add dried cranberries to the pear mixture) and transfer to sterilized glass jars. Screw on the lids and turn upside down while the compote is still warm. The pressure of the compote while cooling will seal the jars ready to store. Alternatively, set aside.

Preheat the oven to 150°C (300°F) Gas 2.

For the granola, mix all the ingredients together in a large mixing bowl so that all the nuts and seeds are coated with maple syrup and cinnamon. Spread the mixture onto the prepared baking sheet and bake in the preheated oven for 10–15 minutes or until golden and toasty.

Remove from the oven and set aside to cool. The mixture will crisp up as it cools. Serve immediately with the pear and cranberry compote or store in an airtight container for up to 1 week.

spiced sweet potato porridge

Sweet potato is the perfect breakfast ingredient because it is a slow-releasing carbohydrate, and the cinnamon here adds sweetness without adding sugar.

200 ml/¾ cup almond milk (or other Paleo milk of choice, see page 11)

2 cinnamon sticks (or 1 teaspoon ground cinnamon), plus extra ground to serve

10 cardamom pods

2 tablespoons pure maple syrup (optional)

150 g/1 cup grated sweet potato

a small handful of mixed nuts and sultanas/golden raisins

1 banana, sliced

SERVES 2

Put the almond milk, cinnamon, cardamom pods and maple syrup, if using, in a saucepan set over medium heat and bring to a gentle simmer. Turn the heat right down so that the milk stays warm and the flavours can infuse for at least 10 minutes. Turn off the heat and cool completely before straining into a jug/pitcher using a fine-mesh sieve/strainer. You could prepare this in advance and store the infused milk in the fridge so it's ready for you to use when required.

Return the infused milk to the pan and bring to a gentle simmer. Add the grated sweet potato and cook for 15–20 minutes, stirring often, or until the potato has softened. Add the nuts and sultanas/golden raisins and stir through.

Pour into your favourite porridge bowl (porridge is such a comforting thing you should take steps to savour it), top with a little sliced banana and, if you're a cinnamon-lover like me, sprinkle with a little ground cinnamon. Enjoy!

choc-ola

Enjoy this chocolatey version of 'granola' for breakfast on an indulgent day with coconut milk, nut milk or coconut yogurt. It's also great as an on-the-go snack.

150 g/1⅓ cups mixed nuts

50 g/⅓ cup mixed seeds

2 tablespoons unsweetened cocoa powder

¾ tablespoon coconut oil

2 tablespoons Sweet Freedom fruit syrup (liquid sweetener), honey or maple syrup

2 tablespoons each of cocoa or cacao nibs and desiccated/shredded coconut

a baking sheet lined with baking parchment

SERVES 4

Preheat the oven to 150°C (300°F) Gas 2.

Mix the nuts and seeds together and spread onto the prepared baking sheet. Bake in the preheated oven for 7 minutes.

Remove from the oven and set aside.

In a saucepan set over low heat, mix the cocoa powder, coconut oil and fruit syrup. Stir to combine. Mix the roasted nuts and seeds into the cocoa mixture so that they are all covered and spread back onto the baking sheet. Roast for a further 5–7 minutes, or until golden and crisp.

Add the cocoa nibs and desiccated/shredded coconut for the last 2 minutes of cooking time. Turn off the oven, leave the door slightly ajar and leave the granola in there to cool.

Once completely cool, serve or store in an airtight container for up to 1 week.

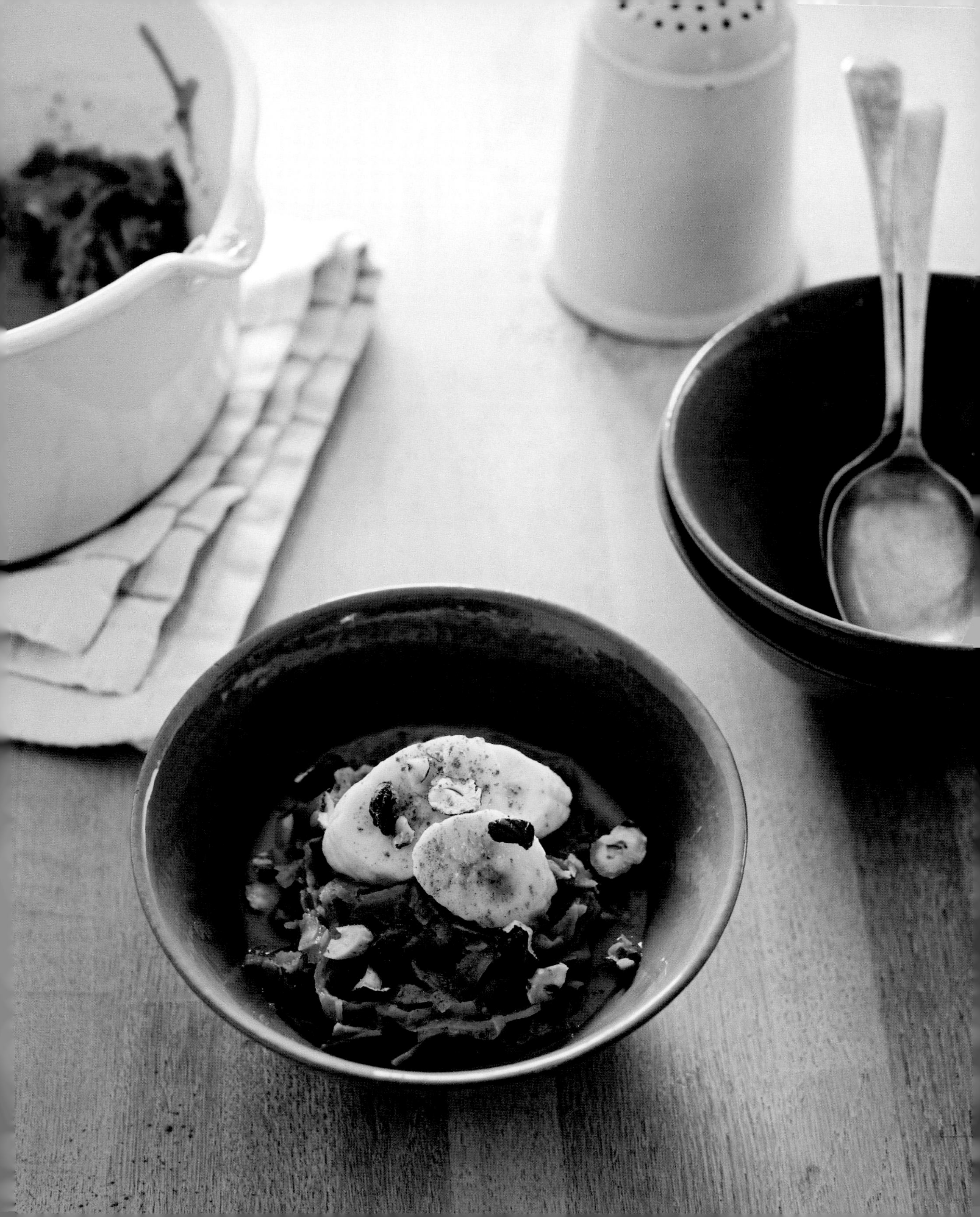

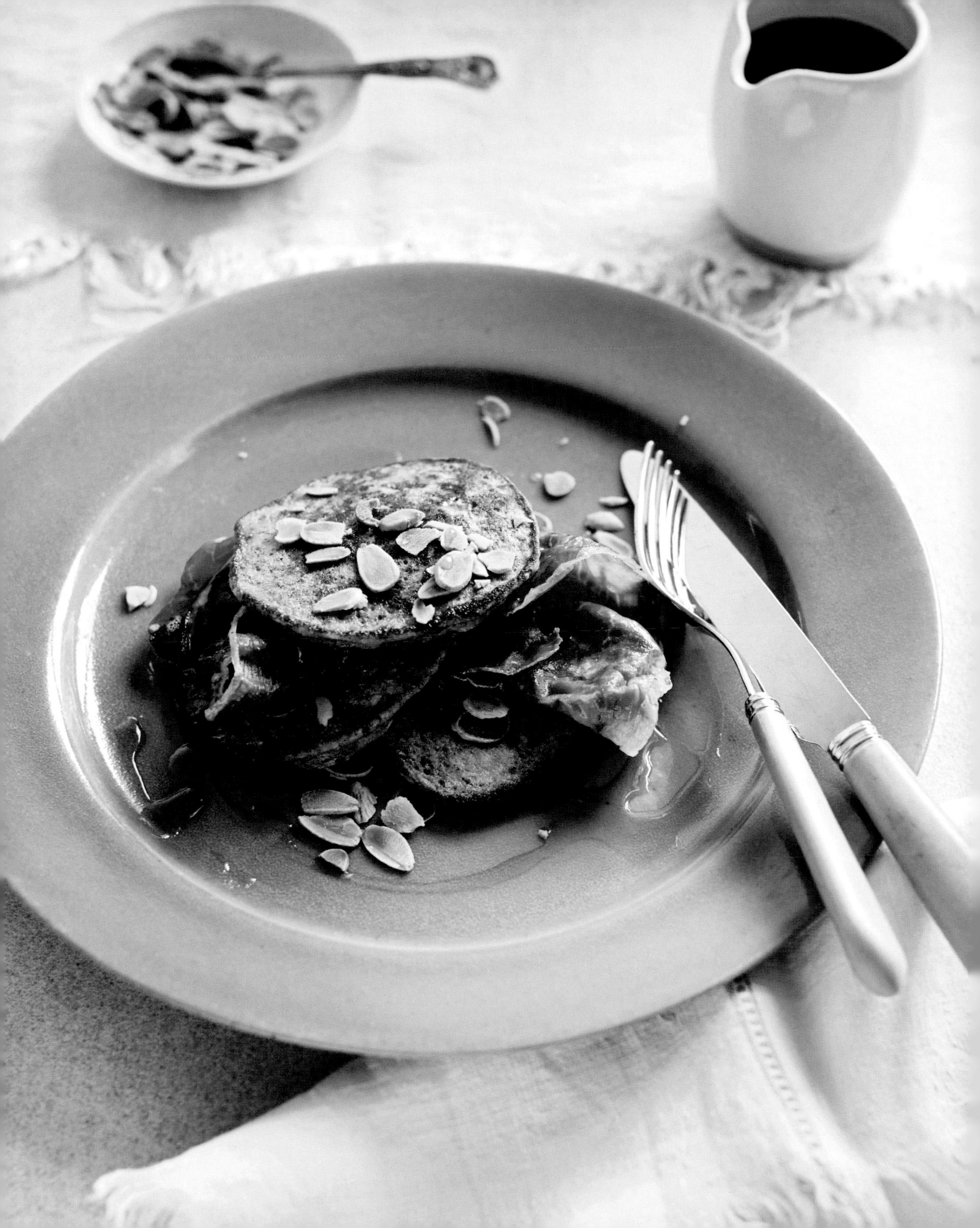

banana pancakes with crispy parma ham

Pancakes are not just for Shrove Tuesday. They are the perfect weekend breakfast with a hit of sweet and savoury to set your taste buds alight. When I worked at the Pure Taste restaurant in London, we used to have Paleo waffles or pancakes with bacon and maple syrup before starting a shift and I've been obsessed ever since!

2 bananas, mashed

2 eggs

1 teaspoon vanilla bean paste (or the seeds from 1 vanilla pod/bean)

1 teaspoon ground cinnamon

2 tablespoons vanilla protein powder (I use SunWarrior®)

1 tablespoon chia seeds

coconut oil (or coconut butter), for frying

to serve

Parma ham

pure maple syrup

flaked/slivered almonds

MAKES 6 PANCAKES AND SERVES 2

Mix all of the ingredients together well in a large mixing bowl and set aside for 10–15 minutes so the chia seeds can start to do their thing – they'll plump up and turn a little gelatinous when in contact with any moisture and adding them here helps to thicken the batter.

Set a non-stick frying pan/skillet over low–medium heat and add a little coconut oil or coconut butter. I find cooking these pancakes over low–medium heat keeps them soft and springy. However, always make sure the pan is heated before adding the batter or the pancakes won't hold their shape and will become flat.

You will need to cook the pancakes in batches of two or three. Pour even spoonfuls of the batter into the pan and when the bubbles start to form on top, they should be ready to flip. Turn over using a spatula and cook the other side of each pancake.

Remove from the pan, turn up the heat and crisp up the Parma ham.

Serve the pancakes in stacks with a drizzle of maple syrup, a sprinkle of flaked/slivered almonds and topped with crispy Parma ham. Enjoy.

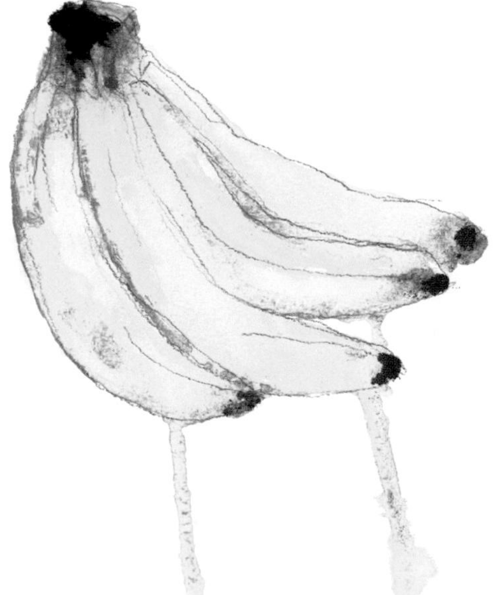

smoked salmon big breakfast

My dad has always made the best salmon weekend brunch. It's one thing I do truly miss from home. Soft-boiled/cooked eggs, crème fraîche, bagels, smoked salmon, vine tomatoes, fresh chives. It's easy enough to sit at the table and avoid the crème fraîche and bagels, but sometimes eggs, salmon and tomatoes on their own just don't cut it. So here's my Paleo blini adaptation – no longer will I suffer food envy!

coconut butter or oil, for frying

225 g/8 oz. vine cherry tomatoes (usually packaged on 2 vines – cut in half for individual portions)

1 large ripe avocado, sliced

1 lemon, cut into wedges

250 g/9 oz. smoked salmon

lumpfish caviar, to serve (optional – if you want to be a bit fancy)

blini batter

60 g/2/3 cup ground almonds

40 g/1/3 cup arrowroot

1 teaspoon baking powder

2 eggs, separated

200 ml/3/4 cup hemp milk (or other Paleo milk of choice, see page 11)

1 tablespoon chopped fresh dill, plus extra to garnish

1 tablespoon chopped fresh parsley

1 tablespoon chopped fresh chives, plus extra to garnish

salt and black pepper, to season

SERVES 4

First, prepare the blini batter. Mix the ground almonds, arrowroot and baking powder together in a large mixing bowl. Make a well in the centre and add the egg yolks and hemp milk. Whisk together slowly to avoid any lumps. Add the herbs and mix in with a fork – they just stick to the whisk if you continue to whisk in. Season well and set aside.

Whisk the egg whites in a separate, clean glass or stainless steel mixing bowl to soft peaks. Fold the egg whites into the batter and rest for 10 minutes.

Set a non-stick frying pan/skillet over low–medium heat, and use a small amount of oil (preferably coconut butter or coconut oil). You will have to cook the blinis in batches – I tend to make enough to allow 2 per person. Pour a little batter into the pan and leave until little bubbles form on the top of each blini. Flip over with a spatula and cook on the other side. Keep warm while you cook the rest of the batter in the same way.

Set another pan with a little oil over medium heat to cook the vine tomatoes. Add the tomatoes (on their vines) to the pan and cook for 3–4 minutes until the bottoms blacken and caramelize. Remove from the heat and set aside.

When ready to serve, top each blini with avocado slices – I tend to slightly squash the avo beforehand, that way you have some smooth parts and some chunky bits. Squeeze with a little lemon to stop it from discolouring, then add slices of smoked salmon on top. Spoon the lumpfish caviar over the top (if using) and arrange the tomatoes on the plate. Finish with a grind of black pepper, a pinch of salt if required, a few sprigs of fresh dill and a few snipped fresh chives.

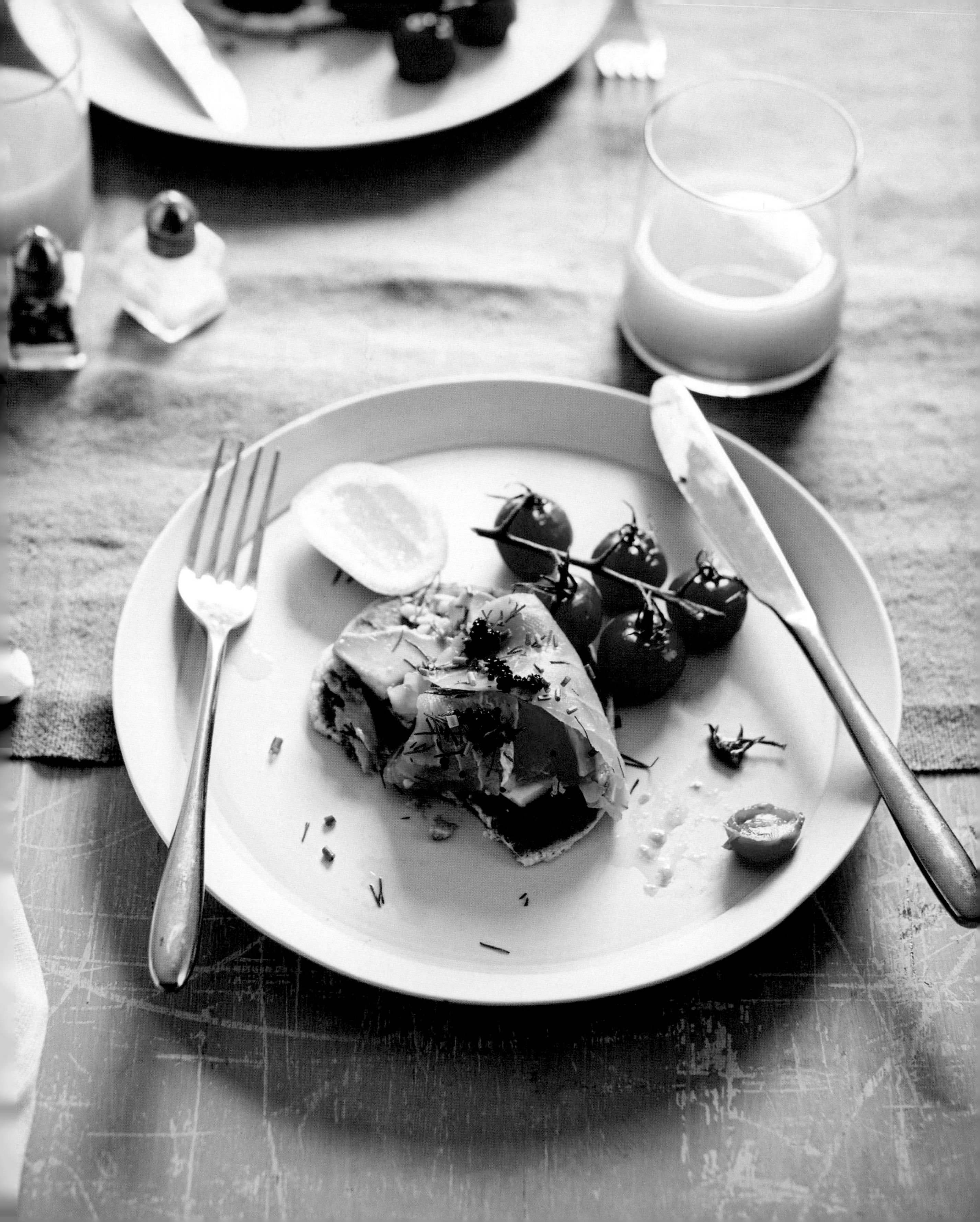

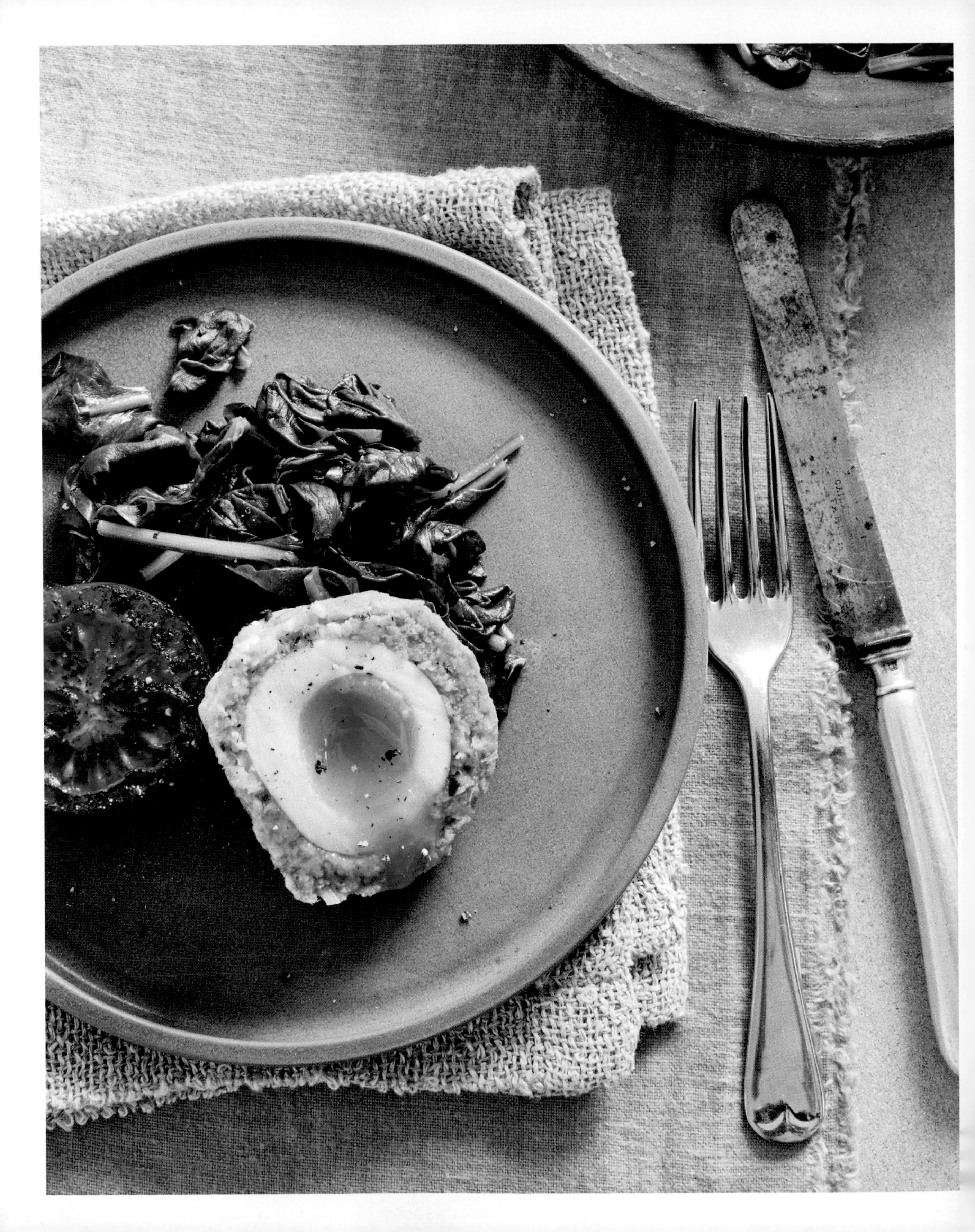

riceless breakfast kedgeree eggs

Swap your fry-up for something different with these breakfast eggs! A spicy coating is wrapped around soft-boiled/cooked eggs and baked to emulate Scotch eggs with the sausage replaced by a flaked fish with a mild curry flavour. Serve with tomatoes and spinach for a larger meal or pack up and take an egg with you for breakfast on-the-run. The sweet potato in the coating helps to bind the mixture.

6 eggs

a bunch of spring onions/ scallions

350 g/12 oz. skinless undyed smoked haddock

2½ teaspoons medium curry powder

½ teaspoon dried chilli/hot red pepper flakes

1½ teaspoons ground turmeric

70 g/⅓ cup cooked sweet potato (optional)

6 medium tomatoes, halved

olive oil, to drizzle (optional)

2–3 large handfuls of spinach

salt and black pepper, to season

a baking sheet lined with baking parchment

MAKES 6 EGGS AND SERVES 6–12 DEPENDING ON WHETHER YOU SERVE THEM HALVED OR WHOLE

Preheat the oven to 170°C (325°F) Gas 3.

Bring a saucepan of water to the boil over medium heat.

Once the water is boiling, gently lower the eggs in and continue to boil for 5 minutes. Lift the eggs out using a slotted spoon and transfer to a bowl of iced water to suspend the cooking for a soft-boiled/cooked egg. If you don't like a runny yolk cook the eggs for longer (1–2 minutes). Once cool, carefully peel the eggs.

Top and tail the spring onions/scallions so you are left with just the middle section, then roughly chop.

Put the haddock, spring onions/scallions, curry powder, chilli/hot red pepper flakes, turmeric and cooked sweet potato (if using) into a food processor and pulse to combine. Process until you have a smooth paste, then scoop the mixture into a mixing bowl.

Form the haddock mixture into 6 patties and lay a patty in one hand. Place a peeled boiled/cooked egg into the middle and wrap the mixture around it. Make sure there are no gaps and set on the prepared baking sheet. Repeat with the remaining patties and eggs. Cook in the preheated oven for 10 minutes.

Meanwhile, grill/broil the tomato halves under medium heat of an overhead grill/broiler or in a frying pan/skillet set over medium heat and drizzled with oil. Heat another frying pan/skillet, if not using the grill/broiler for the tomatoes, with a splash of water or oil over medium heat. Add the spinach and cook for 30 seconds–1 minute, just before serving. Season well with salt and pepper.

Remove the eggs from the oven, cut in half and serve with the spinach and tomatoes. Alternatively, store the eggs whole in an airtight container in the fridge for up to 2 days.

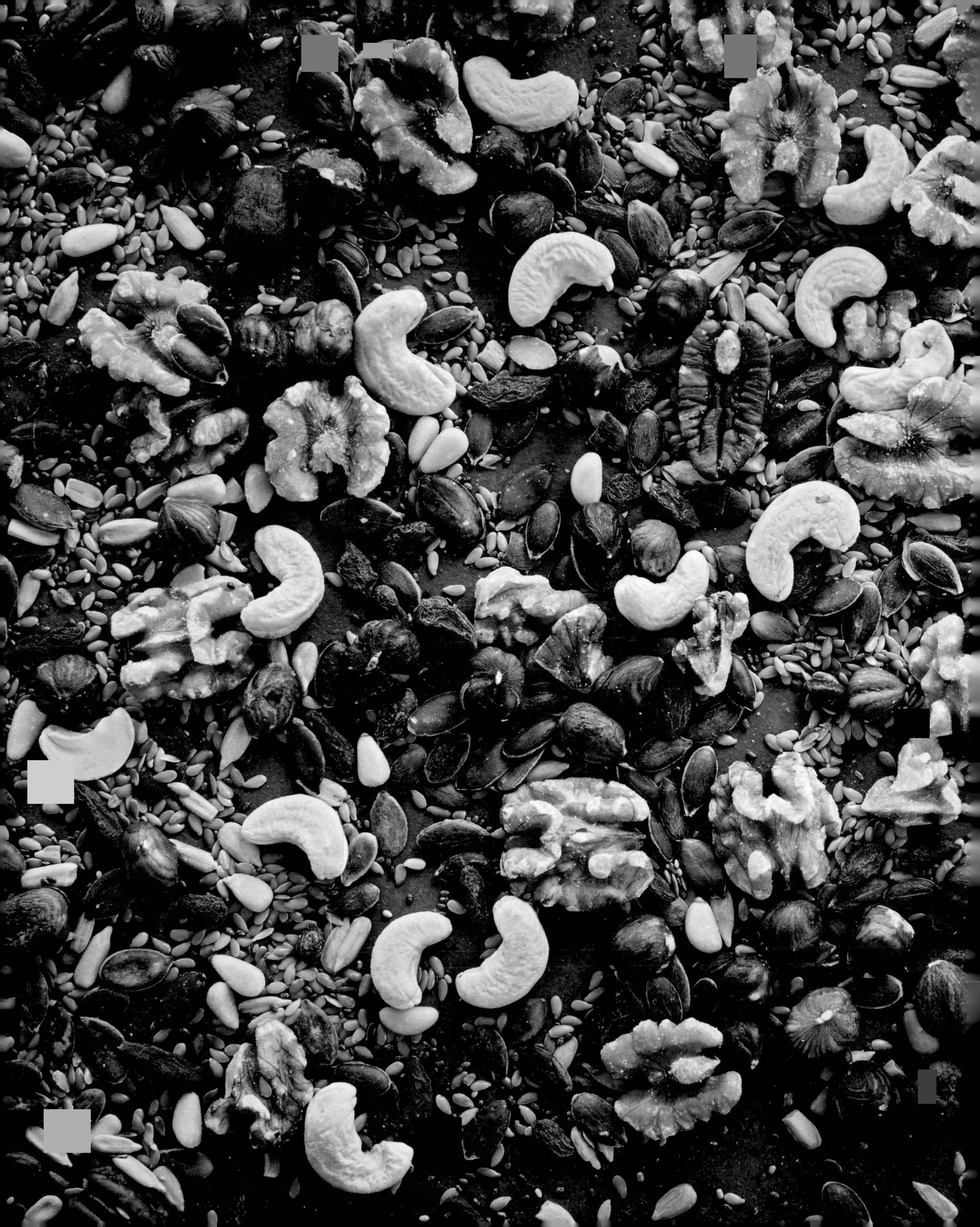

super snacks

I've always been a snacker, whether it's pre-dinner nibbles or an afternoon pick-me-up, I like to have something to keep me going between meals. This chapter is a mix of both sweet and savoury recipes to replace those easy-to-grab chocolate bars and biscuits, crisps and dips.

prawns/shrimp with bacon dip

I use bacon from my uncle's pigs at Hungerford Park farm for this dip – it has quite a thick bit of fat on it, which crisps up amazingly and also produces more excess liquid fat. If you can't get hold of fatty bacon, streaky is a great alternative.

350 g/12 oz. cooked king prawns/jumbo shrimp (tails on), to serve

bacon dip

200 g/7 oz. bacon

3 heaped tablespoons mayonnaise

2 teaspoons harissa paste

1/2 garlic clove, crushed

SERVES 6

Preheat the oven to 200°C (400°F) Gas 6.

For the bacon dip, lay the bacon on a baking pan and bake in the preheated oven for about 10 minutes, or until crisp.

Remove the bacon from the pan – I like to keep the excess fat for other cooking purposes. Finely chop the cooked bacon (or blitz in a food processor) to make a crumb for the dip.

Mix the mayonnaise, harissa paste and crushed garlic clove together and sprinkle with the bacon crumb.

Serve with the cooked king prawns/jumbo shrimp to dip in.

parsnip with avocado dip

I am obsessed with parsnips so often just bung some in the oven when I feel I need a little carb hit. I recommend trying both of the dips on this page with both 'dippers'.

4 parsnips, sliced lengthways

olive oil, to coat

a sprig each of fresh rosemary and tarragon, chopped

salt and black pepper, to season

avocado dip

a handful each of fresh watercress, spinach and rocket/arugula

80 g/2/3 cup cashew nuts

freshly squeezed juice of 1/2 lemon

1/2–1 garlic clove

avocado oil, to drizzle

1/2 avocado

SERVES 6

Preheat the oven to 180°C (350°F) Gas 4.

Coat the parsnips in a little olive oil and sprinkle with the herbs and season with salt and pepper.

Spread the parsnips out on the prepared baking sheet and bake in the preheated oven for 10 minutes, or until golden and slightly crisp – the time will vary depending on the thickness of the parsnips and how much oil you use.

For the avocado dip, blitz all the ingredients except the avocado oil and avocado in a food processor or bash in a large pestle and mortar. Add enough oil to make it a smooth dip similar in consistency to a pesto. Add the avocado and mash to combine.

Season with salt and pepper and serve with the cooked parsnips to dip in.

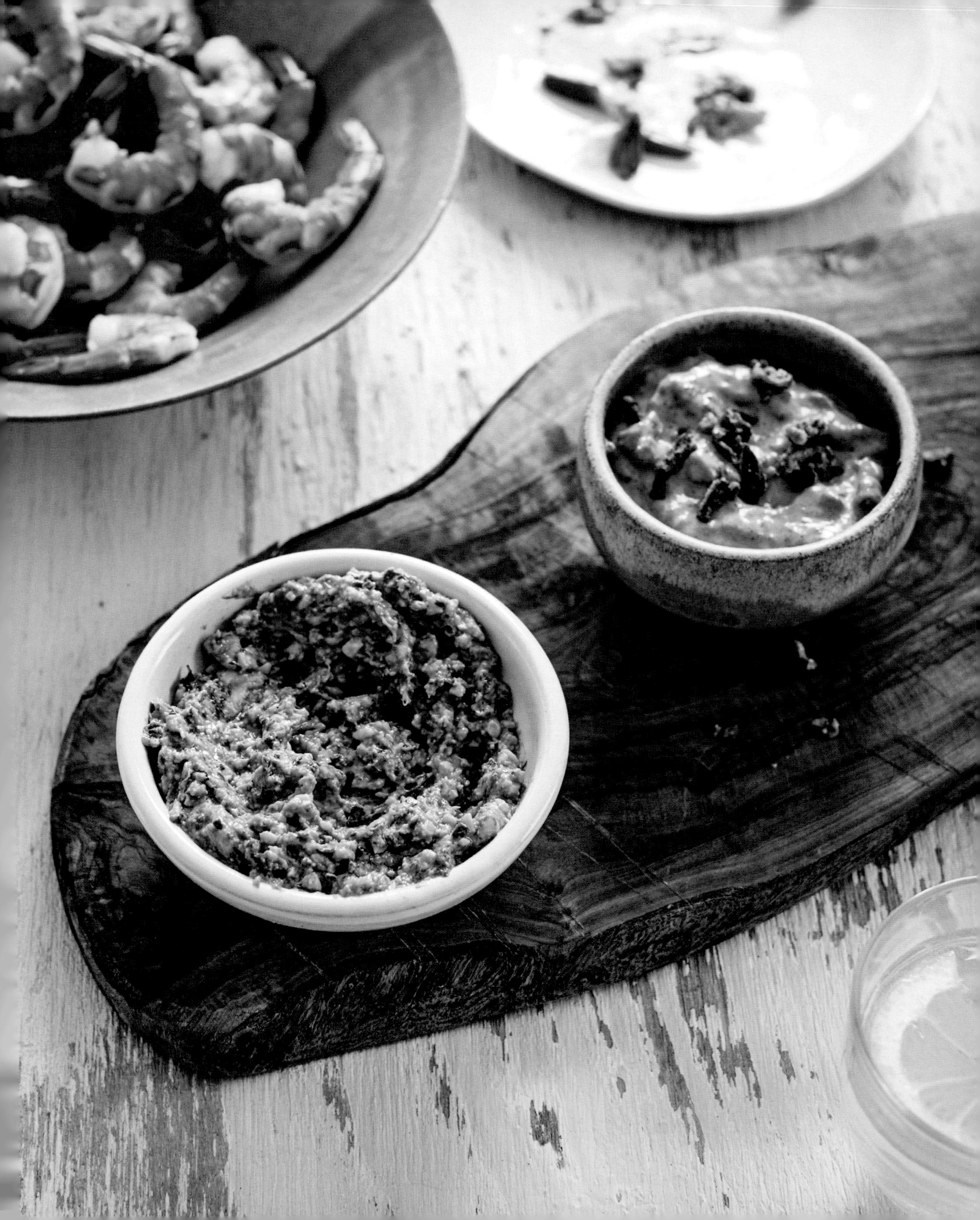

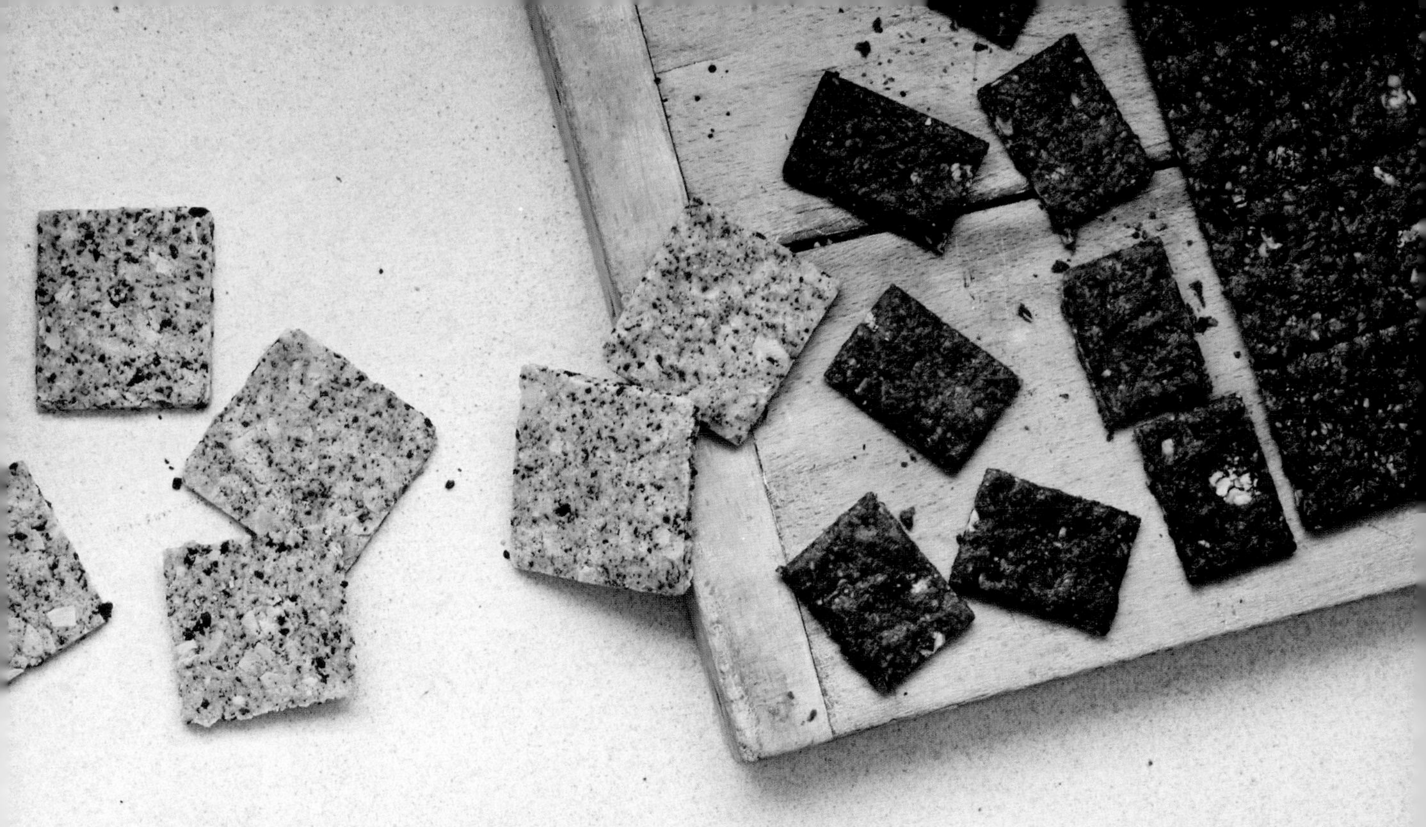

When you need a quick snack, these are great as an alternative to wheat crackers or potato crisps. One was created for my cousin, who owns The Wheatsheaf pub in Wiltshire. He has taught me to be bold with flavours. I raised an eyebrow when he asked me to make a coffee and almond cracker but it really works!

the Ol' Wheatsheaf cracker

130 g/1 1/3 cup ground almonds
50 g/2/3 cup flaked/slivered almonds
a pinch of salt
25 g/1 3/4 tablespoons (or 1 espresso cup) coffee beans, ground
1–1 1/2 egg whites
olive oil, to drizzle
sea salt flakes, to sprinkle

MAKES ABOUT 20

Preheat the oven to 160°C (325°F) Gas 3.

Mix both types of almonds together with a pinch of salt in a large mixing bowl. Break the flaked/slivered almonds up a little so they aren't whole pieces. Add the ground coffee and stir through. Add 1 egg white to bind the mixture. Use your hands to form it into a ball, and if it isn't binding properly add extra white.

Transfer the dough to a sheet of baking parchment and press into a rectangle shape. Oil a rolling pin and roll out until quite thin (no thicker than 5 mm/ 1/4 inch). Transfer to a baking sheet and score the dough to your desired size. Drizzle a little olive oil over the top and sprinkle with sea salt flakes.

Bake in the preheated oven for 8–10 minutes. Remove from the oven. If the biscuits are still a little soft, carefully cut along the scores, turn the heat up to 200°C (400°F) Gas 6 and bake for another 1–2 minutes, or until crisp and golden. Remove from the oven and serve.

apricot kernel thins

50 g/$^{1}/_{3}$ cup apricot kernels (available at health food stores or online)

3 heaped tablespoons apricot kernel butter (available at health food stores or online)

1$^{1}/_{2}$ tablespoons liquid coconut aminos

MAKES 28

Preheat the oven to 150°C (300°F) Gas 2.

Blitz the apricot kernels in a food processor until they break down to a crumb.

Add the rest of the ingredients and blitz until well combined.

Tip out the mixture and roll out thinly into a rectangle between two sheets of baking parchment. It really doesn't need to be any thicker than a couple of millimetres or $^{1}/_{8}$ inch.

Remove the top layer of baking parchment. Score with a sharp knife or a pizza cutter – I score mine into 7 x 4-cm/3 x 1$^{1}/_{2}$-inch rectangles as I like quite small crackers, they are thins after all. Transfer the thins on the baking parchment onto a flat baking sheet without a rim, or if you don't have one then just turn over a regular baking sheet and use upside down – just be careful the baking parchment doesn't slide off (if you have a high-powered fan oven you may need to weigh it down).

Bake in the preheated oven for 5–7 minutes, turn the heat down to 140°C (275°F) Gas 1 and bake for a further 3–5 minutes or until golden.

Remove from the oven and the thins will naturally crisp as they cool.

crispy kale

a bunch of kale

salt and black pepper, to season

a baking sheet lined with baking parchment

SERVES 2–4

Preheat the oven to 160°C (325°F) Gas 3.

Spread the kale out on the prepared baking sheet, sprinkle over salt and pepper, and bake in the preheated oven for 10–15 minutes, or until crisp.

Remove from the oven, leave to cool and enjoy. You can store any leftover kale in an airtight container for up to 2 days.

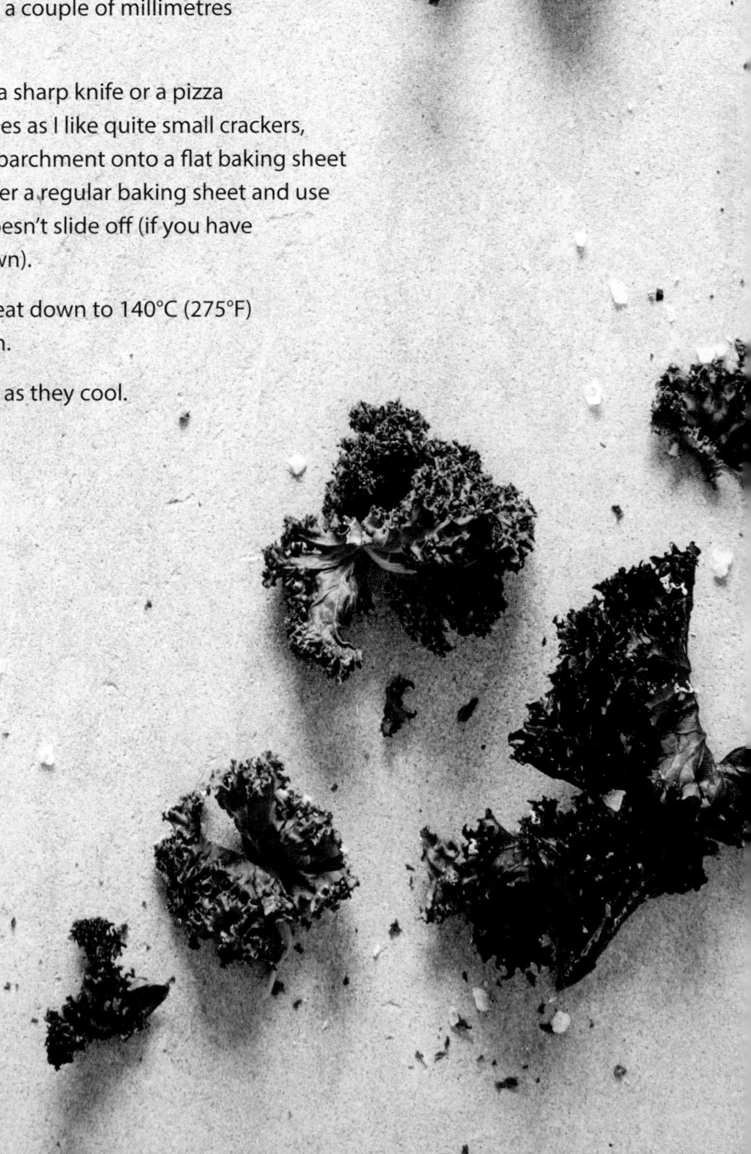

Thai-spiced cashews

You know those bowls of peanuts everyone lays out to nibble on in pubs or at parties, well I never quite trust them. They are usually completely overloaded with sugar and salt and other nonsense. These Thai-spiced cashews are a much cleaner alternative. Use this technique with others nuts and spices and you can have your own unique nut mix going on.

400 g/3½ cups cashew nuts

6–8 teaspoons Thai seven-spice mix, to taste

1–2 egg whites

a baking sheet lined with baking parchment

SERVES 6–8

Preheat the oven to 110°C (225°F) Gas ¼.

Mix together the nuts and spice mix. Add a small amount of the egg white (this is a little trick from my cousin's kitchen – the egg white is just used to bind the spice onto the nut).

Spread the coated nuts out on the prepared baking sheet and bake in the preheated oven for 15 minutes. Check and give the nuts a little shake to make sure they aren't stuck together or to the baking parchment. Turn up the heat to 150°C (300°F) Gas 2 and leave another few minutes until they turn golden.

Remove from the oven, leave to cool and enjoy. You can store any leftover nuts in an airtight container for 3–5 days.

mummy's pumpkin and sunflower seeds

These take me way back to my childhood when my mum used to make us toasted seeds to snack on. She used soy sauce then, however I found the perfect Paleo alternative in liquid coconut aminos, which isn't too dissimilar in taste to the original.

200 g/1½ cups pumpkin seeds

200 g/1½ cups sunflower seeds

liquid coconut aminos, to taste

a baking sheet lined with baking parchment

SERVES 6

Preheat the oven to 160°C (325°F) Gas 3.

I always start by lightly toasting the seeds in a dry non-stick frying pan/skillet over medium heat first.

Transfer the seeds to the prepared baking sheet and drizzle with liquid coconut aminos. The ratio of seeds to liquid aminos is entirely up to you – you can double, triple, quadruple the amount of seeds used here if you want to make a big batch. You want enough liquid aminos to lightly coat the seeds – the more you use the stronger the salt flavour.

Bake in the preheated oven for 4 minutes, or until nice and toasty.

Remove from the oven, leave to cool and enjoy. You can store any leftover seeds in an airtight container for 3–5 days.

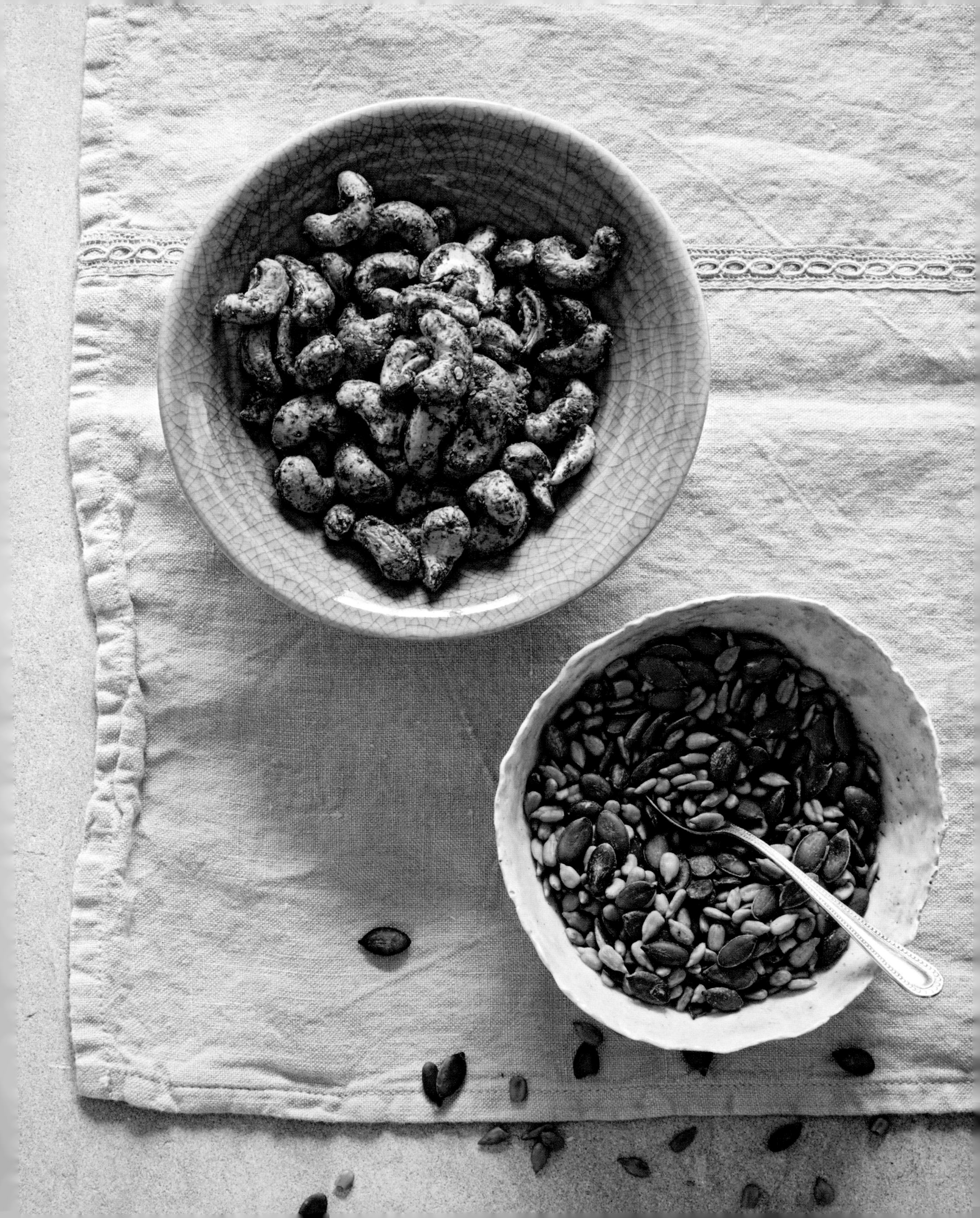

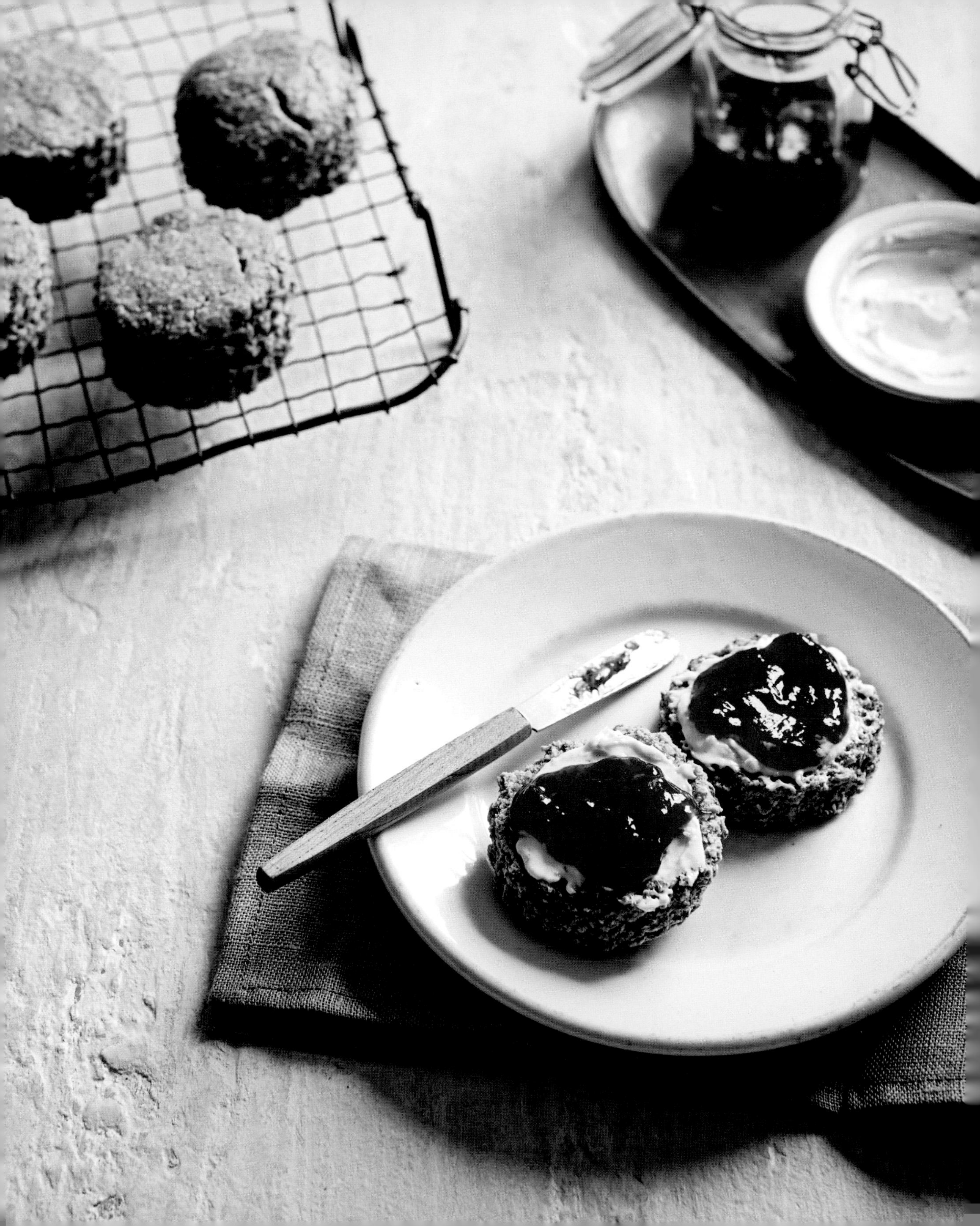

sweet potato scones

I know you might read this recipe, see oats and think I'm breaking the rules. Grains are one of those no-goes on this thing we call 'Paleo', but what is Paleo to me is listening to my body. For me, gluten-free oats are fine but you could use a Paleo flour if you want to.

250 g/2½ cups gluten-free oats

1½ tablespoons xylitol

1 teaspoon ground cinnamon

1 egg, beaten, plus extra for glazing

1 tablespoon freshly squeezed lemon juice

2 tablespoons melted coconut oil

2 tablespoons almond (or coconut) milk

50 g/¼ cup cooked sweet potato (see Note)

½ teaspoon bicarbonate of/ baking soda

½ teaspoon apple cider vinegar

to serve

preserve of your choice (pages 12–13)

Paleo butter (or coconut cream)

a high-powered blender (I use a NutriBullet)

a round cookie cutter

a baking sheet lined with baking parchment

MAKES 4–6

Preheat the oven to 180°C (350°F) Gas 4.

Blitz the oats in a high-powered blender so they form a flour. Set a small amount aside for dusting the surface and cookie cutter when cutting out.

Add the xylitol and cinnamon to the oat flour and blitz again. Transfer the mixture to a large mixing bowl. Make a well in the centre, add the beaten egg, lemon juice, coconut oil and almond milk. Using a wooden spoon, slowly mix the wet ingredients into the dry, until everything is combined. The mix will look a bit like a separated dough. Add the cooked sweet potato. At this point I use my hands to help combine all the ingredients, you don't want to over work the mix but don't be afraid to squish it all together – it will form a sort of dough.

In a separate small bowl, mix the bicarbonate of/baking soda and apple cider vinegar together, it will fizz up but just add it to your dough straight away. Mix to combine.

Dust a clean work surface with the reserved oat flour and lightly roll out the dough to a thickness of about 2.5–5 cm/1–2 inches. Stamp out rounds using the cookie cutter (dust with a little oat flour if it sticks). Arrange the rounds on the prepared baking sheet, glaze with the beaten egg and bake for 15 minutes.

Remove from the oven and serve with a preserve of your choice and butter or coconut cream.

Note: The ideal way to use cooked sweet potato for baking is to have already baked it and let it cool. This can be done in advance and the potato can be stored in the fridge. You can cook the sweet potato just before you bake the scones but it needs time to cool down properly before you use it. Simply pop a sweet potato in a preheated oven at 160°C (325°F) Gas 3, no fuss. I tend to cook them for 45 minutes–1 hour depending on the size of the potato. All you want is for it to be soft and cooked through. If you cook it at a lower temperature there is no need for you to pierce the potato as you won't need to worry about it exploding all over the oven.

salmon eggs with herbed mayo

These salmon eggs are great for snacking after a workout as they will satisfy hunger without leaving you feeling too full or bloated. Protein is really important for muscle repair and so these are the ideal snack. Make a batch and store them in the fridge so they are ready for you when you need them.

12 quail's eggs
zest of 1 lemon, plus extra wedges to serve
2 spring onions/scallions, roughly chopped
1 salmon fillet (roughly 160 g/6 oz.)
100 g/3½ oz. smoked salmon
1 teaspoon dried chilli/hot red pepper flakes
1 teaspoon coconut flour
unscented coconut oil, for frying (optional)
salt and black pepper, to season
Herbed Mayo (page 14), to serve

a baking sheet lined with baking parchment

MAKES 12 AND SERVES 4–6

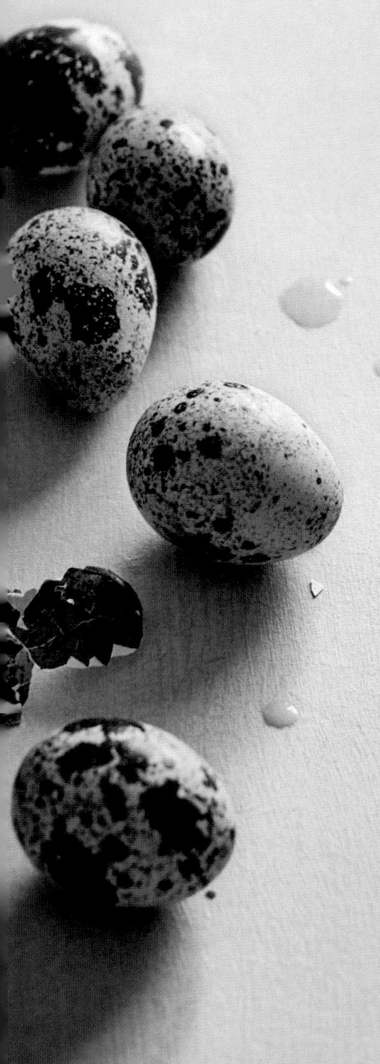

Preheat the oven to 180°C (350°F) Gas 4.

Bring a saucepan of water to the boil over medium heat and, once at a rolling boil, turn down the heat and carefully lower in the eggs. Turn the heat back up to high and cook for 2 minutes 40 seconds (or longer if you prefer and firmer set yolk). Lift the eggs from the water using a slotted spoon and put straight into a bowl of iced water.

Once cold carefully peel eggs. It's best to lightly crack the whole of the shell and dip it back into the water so the shell comes away easily from the white. Drain on paper towels and set aside in a cool place.

Put the lemon zest, spring onions/scallions, salmon fillet and smoked salmon in the bowl of a food processor. Blitz for a few seconds at a time until both types of salmon are well blended. Add the chilli/hot red pepper flakes, season with a little salt and pepper, and blitz again to combine.

Carefully roll each peeled egg in a little coconut flour, just to help the salmon mixture bind around it.

Make 12 patties from the salmon mixture and lay a patty in the palm of one hand. Place a peeled egg into the middle and wrap the mixture around it. Make sure there are no gaps and set on the prepared baking sheet. Repeat.

Bake the eggs in the preheated oven for 6–8 minutes. Alternatively, shallow fry them in a small amount of unscented coconut oil over medium heat, turning occasionally to cook evenly.

Remove from the oven or pan and leave to cool slightly before squeezing over a lemon wedge. I like to cut the eggs in half so that you can see the yolk when you serve them, but you can serve them whole with the herbed mayo on the side for dipping.

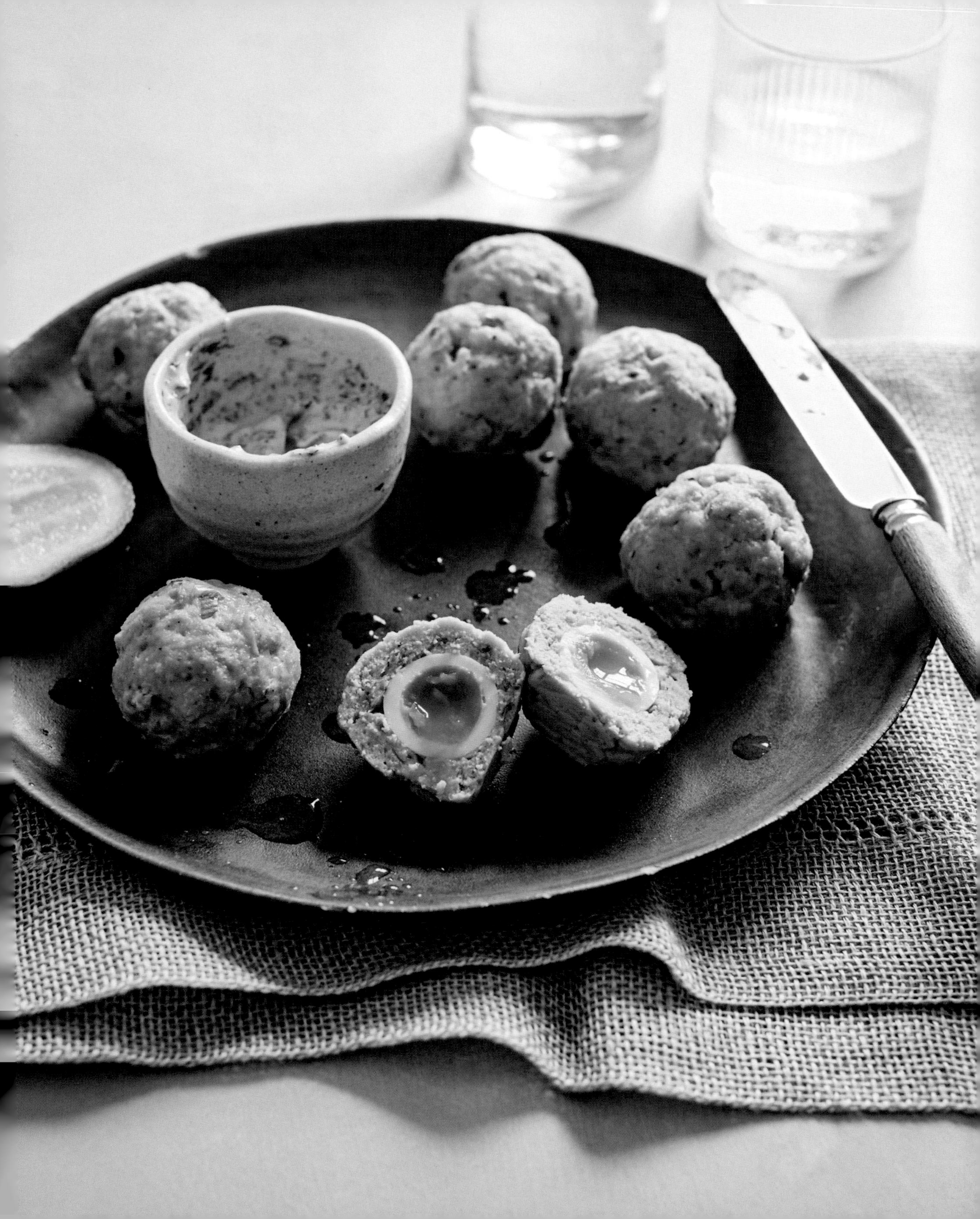

paleo pork pie

A traditional pork pie comprises roughly chopped pork and pork jelly sealed in a pastry case. A Paleo pork pie is the same but all made from scratch and without gluten. I'm not going to sugar-coat it; this is a long-winded process. You can use store-bought gelatine and stock, and lard instead of fat in the pastry, but I think for the best flavour it's great to make each part. Make friends with your butcher who can cut the bone for you to release the marrow.

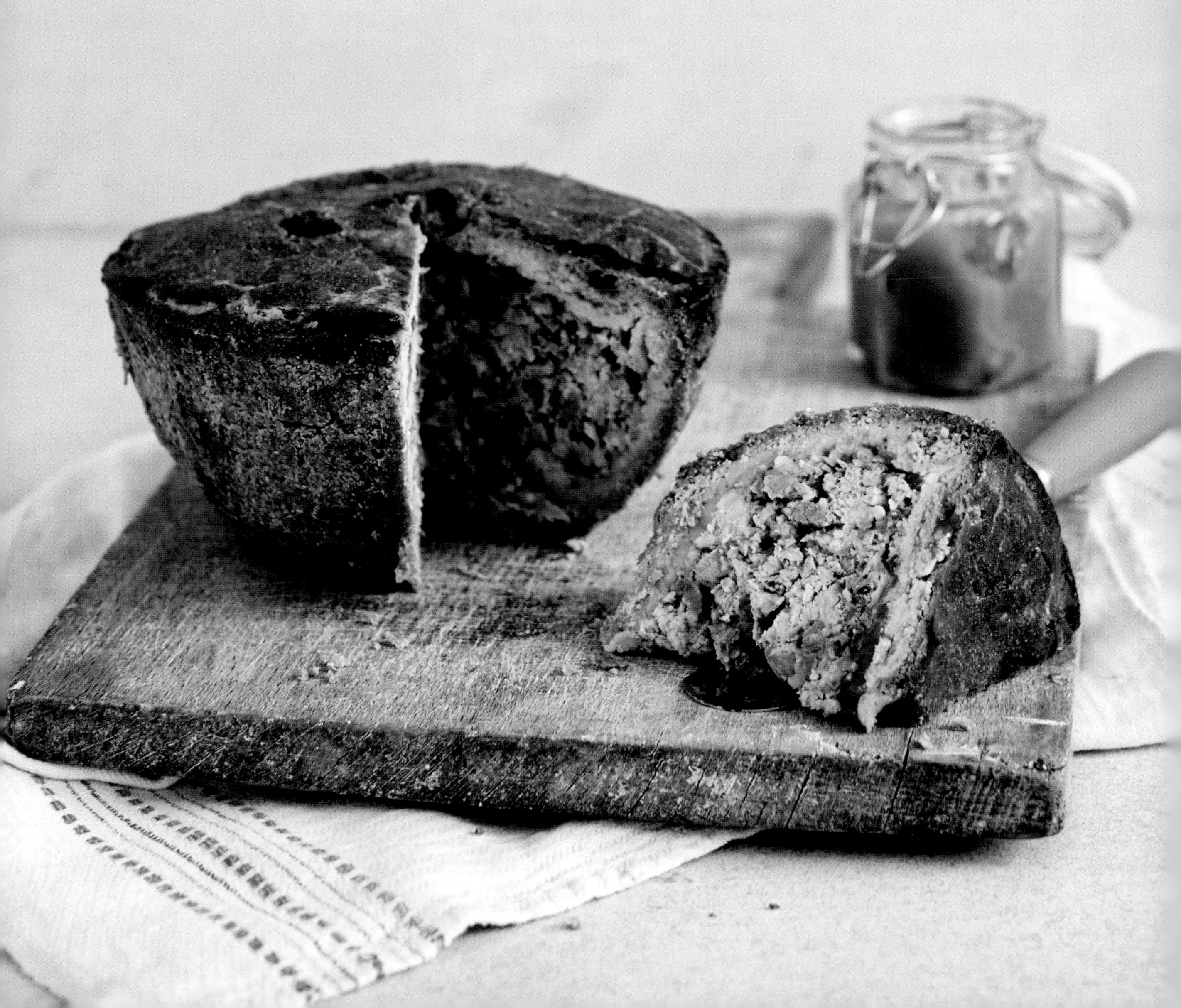

Apple Sauce (page 14), to serve

gelatine

1–2 pig's feet

1 pork bone

1 carrot, roughly chopped

2 celery stalks/ribs, roughly chopped

1 onion, halved

a few springs of fresh sage, rosemary and thyme

1 teaspoon black peppercorns

1 garlic clove

pastry

100 g/1 cup almond flour

85–100 g/scant 1 cup chestnut (or almond) flour

75 g/3/4 cup arrowroot, plus extra for rolling

a pinch of salt

80 g/3 oz. clarified pork fat (see Note)

1 egg, plus 1 beaten egg for glazing

2–4 tablespoons cold water

pork filling

6 juniper berries

8 sage leaves

100 g/scant 1 cup finely diced white onion

1/4 teaspoon ground nutmeg

250 g/9 oz. ground pork

150 g/5 1/2 oz. pork meat, chopped into small pieces

1 tablespoon pork fat, for frying

a deep 500-g/18-oz. capacity baking pan, greased with pork fat or lard

SERVES 6–8

First make the gelatine. In a large saucepan cover all the ingredients in water, cover with a lid and bring to the boil over medium heat and cook for 1–2 hours. For best results, transfer this liquid and the ingredients to a container, cool, seal and set in the fridge overnight, then bring to the boil again the next day, but you could skip this part. Simmer uncovered to reduce the liquid to about 300 ml/1 1/4 cups. Strain the liquid into a jug/pitcher. To check that you have extracted the gelatine content from the bones, put it in the fridge. You may need to skim the top of a fatty layer and beneath that layer it should have set to jelly. You can do this a day or two before making the pork pie as you can store it in the fridge until you are ready to use it, for up to 3 days.

To make the pastry, mix the dry ingredients in a large mixing bowl. Rub in the clarified pork fat. Mix in the egg and 2 tablespoons of cold water. Add a little more water if necessary and form into a ball. Push the pastry ball into the base of the prepared baking pan and up the sides to a thickness of about 5 mm/ 1/4 inch. Trim away any excess and form into another ball for the pastry top. Put the lined pan in the freezer while you prepare the pork filling.

Preheat the oven to 200°C (400°F) Gas 6.

For the pork filling, crush the juniper berries and sage leaves together in a pestle and mortar and set aside. Set a frying pan/skillet over low–medium heat and sauté the onions in the pork fat. Add the ground juniper berries and sage, as well as the nutmeg. When the onions have softened and become clear, remove the pan from the heat and set aside to cool. Once the onion mixture is completely cool, mix with the ground pork and chopped pork meat. Set aside.

Roll out the reserved pastry on a surface lightly dusted with arrowroot. Fill the chilled pastry case with the pork filling. Brush a little beaten egg around the edge and lay the pastry top over. Press the edges together to seal, then cut a hole in the top. Brush the beaten egg over the top.

Bake in the preheated oven for 20 minutes, turn the heat down to 160°C (325°F) Gas 3 and bake for 35–45 minutes. If for some reason the pastry looks like it is cracking during the cooking process, just brush with a little extra beaten egg.

Remove the pie from the oven and leave to cool. Meanwhile, melt the gelatine in a saucepan over low heat. The pie doesn't have to be cold but once cooled, use a funnel to pour the melted gelatine into the top of the pie a little at a time. Be patient when pouring in the gelatine – it's finding its way into all the gaps. Set in the fridge for a few hours or overnight, then serve with apple sauce.

Note: To clarify the pork fat, preheat the oven to 200°C (400°F) Gas 6. Put pork fat off-cuts (ask your butcher for these or trim from a piece of pork belly) in a deep baking dish. Cook in the preheated oven for 30–40 minutes, checking every 5–10 minutes and transferring any liquid fat that is released to a heatproof bowl. Once you have collected all the liquid fat, put the bowl in the fridge to solidify the fat. You can store this in a tub in the fridge and use it for other Paleo cooking. Alternatively buy good-quality lard.

fruit buns with honey butter

Hot cross buns are one of my favourite treats and these are a pretty close match. I always eat mine with butter on one side and butter and honey on the other. I buy a local, raw, organic honey made by my uncle's bees kept on Hungerford Park – there is nothing better than knowing where your produce has come from!

100 ml/1/3 cup Sweet Freedom fruit syrup (or maple syrup)

230 ml/1 cup hemp milk (or other Paleo milk of choice, see page 11)

1 1/2 tablespoons fast-action gluten-free yeast

130 g/1 1/3 cup almond flour, plus a little extra for kneading

110 g/1 cup ground almonds

210 g/1 1/2 cups arrowroot

2 teaspoons mixed spice/ apple pie spice

1/2 teaspoon ground cinnamon

1/4 teaspoon ground nutmeg

50 g/5 tablespoons coconut oil (or coconut butter)

a pinch of salt

2 eggs, beaten

85 g/1/2 cup sultanas/golden raisins and 40 g/1/4 cup mixed dried currants and blueberries (I use Urban Fruit)

30 g/2 tablespoons goji berries

Honey Butter, to serve (page 14)

to glaze

1 egg

1 tablespoon palm sugar

a baking sheet, greased with coconut oil and dusted with arrowroot

MAKES 8–10

Mix together 15 ml/1 tablespoon of your sweetener of choice with 60 ml/ 1/4 cup lukewarm hemp milk and the yeast. Set aside in a warm place for 5 minutes to activate the yeast.

Sift together the almond flour, ground almonds and arrowroot into a large mixing bowl. Mix in the spices and rub in the coconut oil with your hands. Mix in the salt and the remainder of the sweetener.

Add the beaten eggs to the hemp milk mixture and stir through.

Make a well in the flour and spice mixture and pour most of the eggy milk mixture into it. Mix well – it should come together to form a soft dough. Add the rest of the milk if required.

Beat for about 1 minute until the dough is smooth. Add the dried fruit and knead in the bowl so the fruit is evenly distributed. Cover with clingfilm/plastic wrap and set in a warm place for 1–1 1/2 hours to rise – it should double in size.

Turn the dough out onto a surface dusted with almond flour. Knead for 1–2 minutes, then divide into 8–10 balls of equal size. Arrange in lines on the prepared baking sheet with a small gap between each. I like to leave just a small gap because it's nice if they join up when they cook so you can tear them to serve.

Beat the egg and palm sugar together to make a glaze and brush over the tops of the buns.

Set in a warm place for about 30 minutes, or until risen a little. Preheat the oven to 220°C (425°F) Gas 7.

Bake in the preheated oven for 5 minutes. Turn the heat down to 200°C (400°F) Gas 6 or 180°C (350°F) Gas 4 depending how fast they are colouring and bake for a further 10–15 minutes until golden. They are ready when there is a hollow sound when you tap the base.

Transfer to a wire rack to cool a little.

Serve hot, toasted or cold, spread with honey butter.

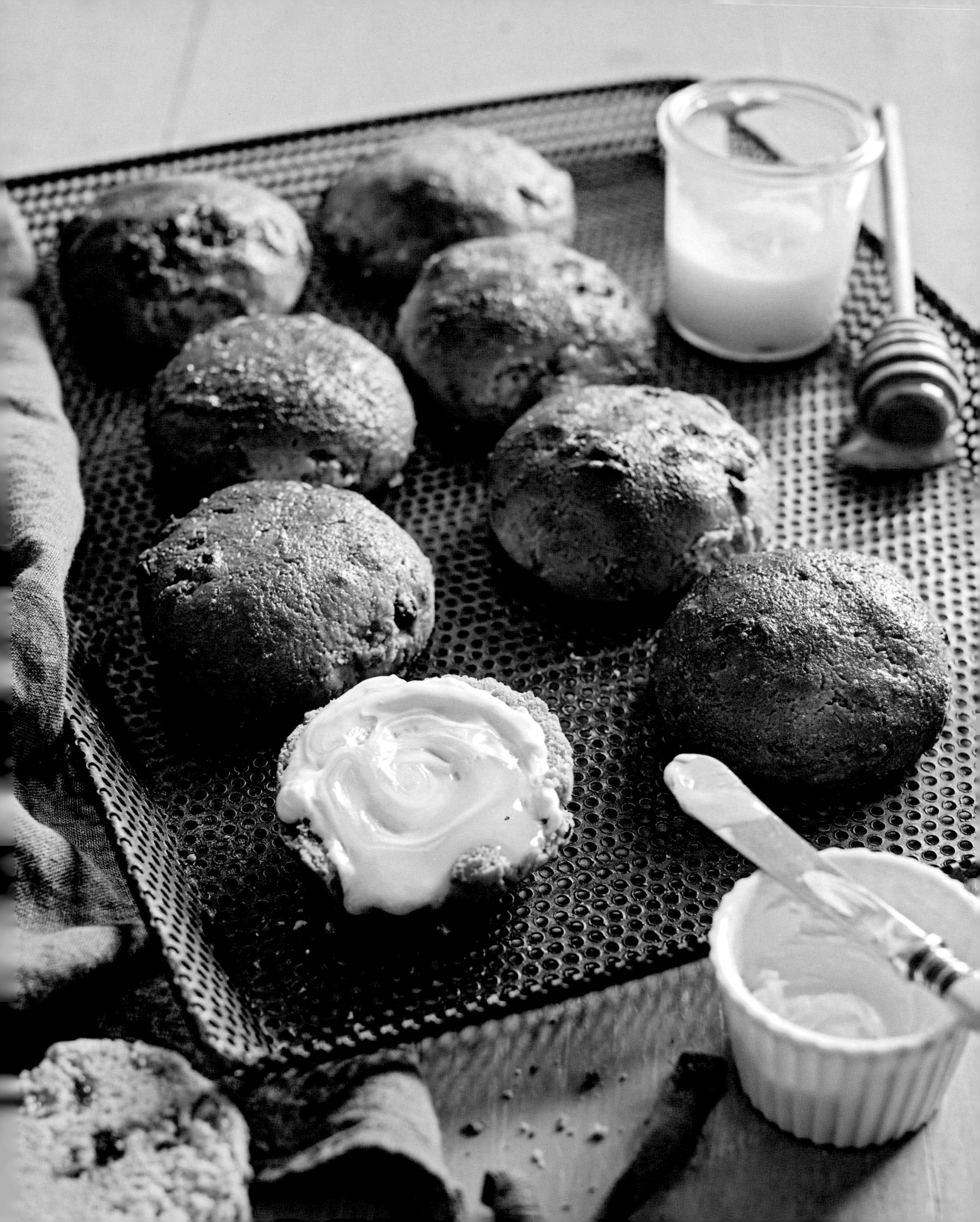

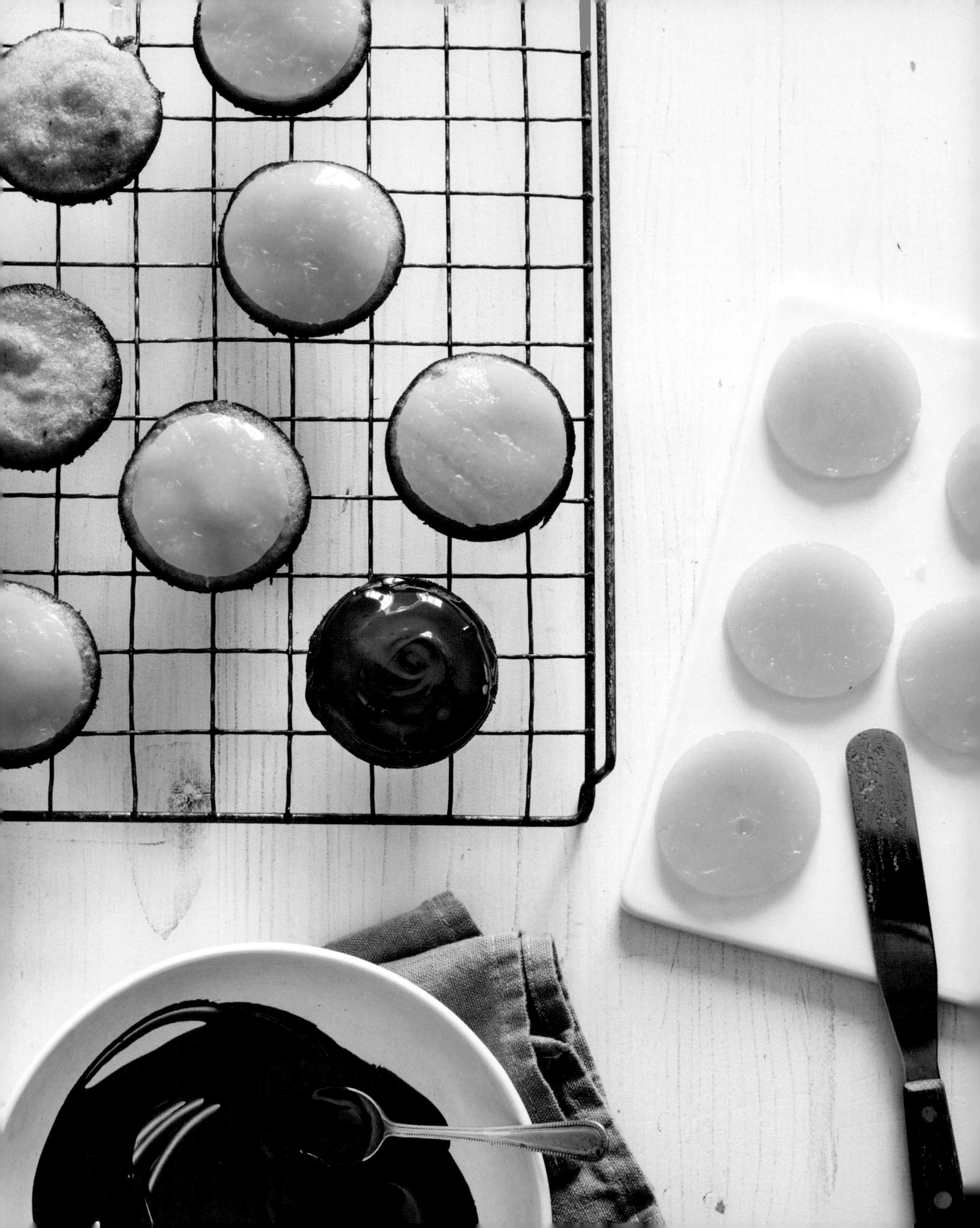

jaffa cakes

A lot of my food inspiration comes from my childhood. My great-grandmother always used to have Jaffa cakes (a small British sponge cake) in the cupboard, and we used to re-enact the 'full moon, half moon, total eclipse' advert, while eating them every time we had one. There are lots of ways you can include treats in a Paleo diet but these are really delightful as a mid-morning snack.

100 g/3½ oz. dairy-free dark/ bittersweet chocolate (I love Willie's Cacao, especially Venezuelan Black)

orange jelly

grated zest of 1 orange

300 ml/1¼ cups freshly squeezed orange juice (or pure orange juice with bits)

12 g/½ oz. grass-fed gelatine (such as Great Lakes)

50 ml/3½ tablespoons boiling water

sponge base

1 egg yolk

85 g/¾ cup plus 1 tablespoon ground almonds

50 g/2½ tablespoons honey

1 teaspoon pure vanilla extract

2 egg whites

a deep baking pan lined with baking parchment or clingfilm/ plastic wrap

a muffin pan, greased with coconut oil

a 5-cm/2-inch cookie cutter

MAKES 12

Start by preparing the orange jelly. Warm the zest and orange juice in a saucepan over medium heat. Dissolve the gelatine in the boiling water in a small bowl stirring constantly. When the orange juice is warmed through but not boiling, slowly add it to the gelatine, stirring constantly.

Set aside to cool slightly, stirring occasionally, then pour into the prepared baking pan to a depth of 5 mm/¼ inch. Refrigerate for at least 3 hours, or until the jelly has set. This mixture makes more than you need, but I find it's helpful having extra jelly at the ready... just in case.

Meanwhile, prepare the sponge base. Preheat the oven to 170°C (325°F) Gas 3.

In a medium mixing bowl, mix together the egg yolk, ground almonds, honey and vanilla. In a separate clean bowl, whisk the egg whites to form soft peaks. Add one spoonful of the egg whites to the almond mixture and stir in to loosen the mixture slightly. Fold in the rest of the egg whites until fully combined. Do not over-mix as you need to keep the air in the egg whites.

Spoon the mixture evenly into the prepared muffin pan and bake in the preheated oven for 15 minutes. Once cooked, remove from the oven and leave to stand for 5 minutes before transferring to a wire rack.

Once the sponge bases are cool and the jelly is set, you need to top the base with jelly. Stamp out rounds of jelly using the cookie cutter. I find the easiest way to transfer the jelly is to lay the sponge bases top-side flat on top of the jelly rounds, then use a flat palette knife to slide underneath the jelly circle, lift off the surface and turn over at the same time.

Once all your jellies are on the bases, melt the chocolate in a heatproof bowl suspended over a saucepan of barely simmering water. Allow the chocolate to cool a little before coating the top of each cake or else it will melt the jelly.

Leave to set and serve or store in an airtight container in the fridge or a cool place so that the jelly and chocolate don't melt for up to 3 days.

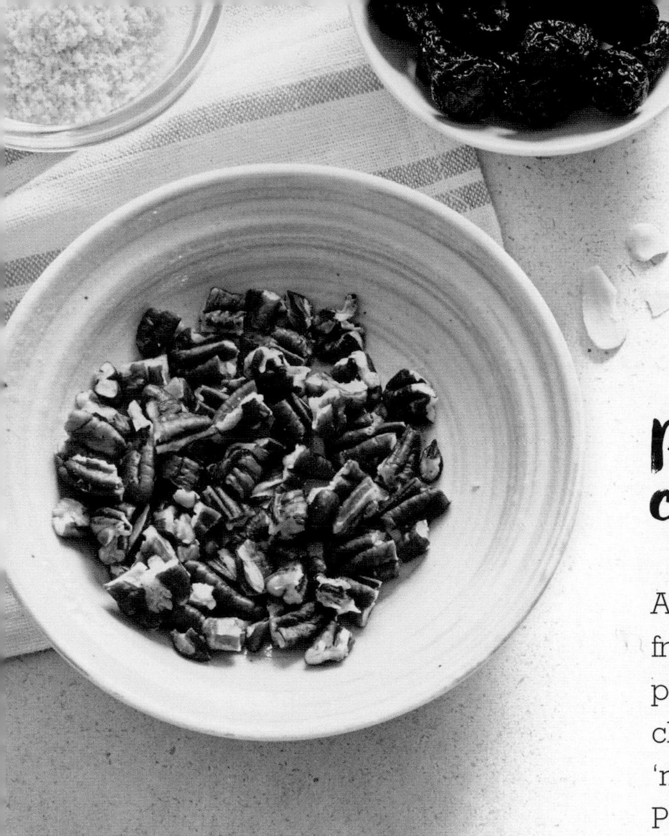

pecan and cherry florentine

A chewy treat made from nuts and dried fruits is perfect for those mid-morning cravings, proving you needn't go without to still eat clean. My step-dad's response to these was, 'mmm, they are very delicious, are they Paleo?' and that is all I can say on that matter.

60 g/½ cup organic dried cherries (I use Urban Fruit)

135 g/1¾ cup flaked/slivered almonds

75 g/¾ cup roughly chopped pecans

35 g/¼ cup ground almonds

30 g/2 tablespoons coconut oil

135 g/1 cup Sweet Freedom fruit syrup

100 g/3½ oz. dairy-free dark/bittersweet chocolate (70% cocoa solids)

2 baking sheets lined with baking parchment

MAKES ABOUT 30

Preheat the oven to 170°C (325°F) Gas 3.

Mix together the dried cherries, flaked/slivered almonds, pecans and ground almonds. Set aside.

Melt together the coconut oil and the fruit syrup in a small pan set over low–medium heat. Bring to a simmer for about 3 minutes until it begins to caramelize. Pour in the fruit and nut mixture. Stir well until fully combined.

Spoon equal amounts of the mixture onto the prepared baking sheets allowing space for spreading. Flatten each spoonful using an oiled back of a spoon. You want to get the mixture as thin and even as possible without pushing it apart.

Bake the Florentines in the preheated oven for 6 minutes or until golden and crisping up. Put the baking sheets onto a wire rack and allow to cool and firm up before lifting off the baking parchment using a palette knife.

Once the Florentines are completely cool, melt the chocolate. Put the chocolate in a heatproof bowl suspended over a pan of barely simmering water. Gently and slowly melt the chocolate. I always remove the chocolate before it is fully melted and stir a little so that it melts evenly and doesn't burn. Brush the chocolate onto the smooth side of the Florentines. Lay them chocolate-side up on a cooling rack and leave to set. You can do a double chocolate layer if you want, or serve as they are.

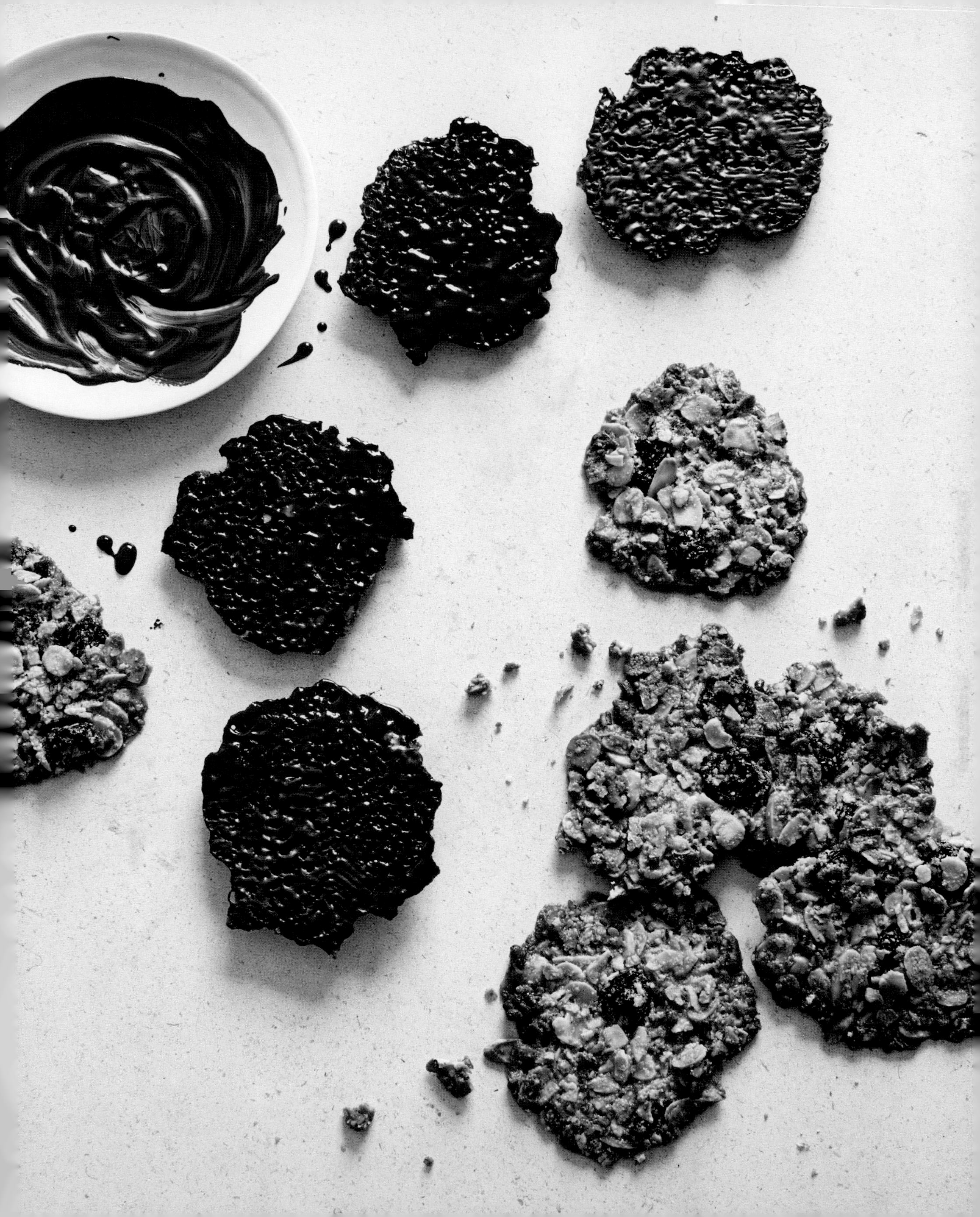

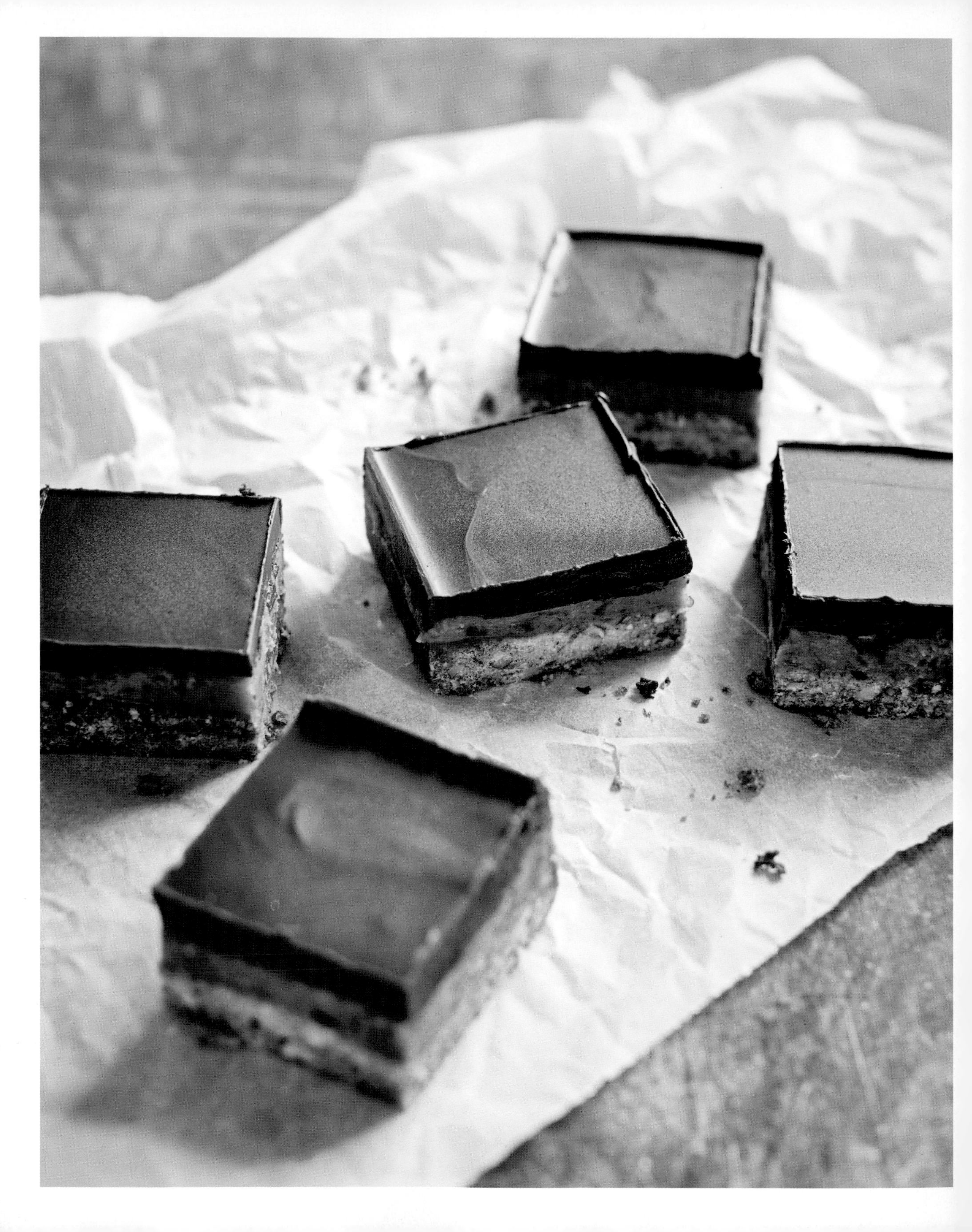

barney's millionaires

My friend Barney made me promise to make him a Paleo millionaire shortbread one day. So, here it is, with a host of his favourite flavours mixed into one delicious treat. I hope you enjoy it as much as he does!

caramel layer

350 g/1 1/3 cup strawberry jam/jelly (I use St. Dalfour)

140 ml/2/3 cup unsweetened almond milk

170 g/3/4 cup coconut butter

40 g/3 tablespoons cacao butter, grated (optional)

base

160 g/1 1/4 cups hazelnuts

135 g/1 1/3 cups almond flour

3/4 teaspoon bicarbonate of/ baking soda

25 g/1 3/4 tablespoons coconut butter, melted

125 g/7 tablespoons honey (or Sweet Freedom fruit syrup)

chocolate layer

75 g/5 1/2 tablespoons coconut butter

15 g/1 tablespoon Sweet Freedom fruit syrup (optional)

300 g/10 1/2 oz. dairy-free dark/bittersweet chocolate, broken into small pieces

a 23-cm/9-inch square deep baking pan lined with baking parchment

MAKES 16

To make the caramel layer, start by mixing the jam/jelly with the almond milk in a saucepan. Set over medium heat and bring to a simmer to melt the jam/jelly. Add the coconut butter and simmer again until it reduces a little. Stir occasionally to combine the coconut butter with the caramel.

Once the strawberry mixture has thickened and is glossy, add the cacao butter and whisk with a fork to ensure everything is well combined. (I add cacao butter because I like the subtle hint of white chocolate flavour it gives the caramel.) Bring to a boil for a few minutes. Once the bubbles slow, remove the pan from the heat and stir occasionally as the caramel cools.

Set aside, but don't let it set through – you need to be able to pour or spoon it over the biscuit bases. Preheat the oven to 160°C (325°F) Gas 3.

To make the base, blitz the hazelnuts in a food processor – alternatively you could use ground hazelnuts but I prefer the texture of skin-on hazelnuts and like to chop a small handful to add to the mixture to add a little crunch.

Mix together the now ground hazelnuts, almond flour and bicarbonate of/ baking soda in a large mixing bowl. Pour in the melted coconut butter and sweetener and stir. Using your hands bring the mixture together and press evenly into the prepared baking pan, making sure the surface is flat and smooth (I use an oiled metal spoon for this). Prick all over with a fork.

Bake in the preheated oven for 10–20 minutes or until golden. The base sometimes puffs up as it bakes but you can flatten it with the back of a metal spoon to keep it flat. Remove the base from the oven and leave to cool in the pan on a wire rack – the base will firm up as it cools. Once the base is cool top with the cooled caramel and smooth over the surface.

To make the chocolate topping, melt coconut butter in a saucepan over low heat, adding the fruit syrup if using. Remove the pan from the heat and add the chocolate. Stir occasionally to melt it. If the chocolate isn't completely melted after 10 minutes return the pan back to very low heat until it does. Stir, then pour on top of caramel. Put in the fridge to set.

Once the chocolate is set, cut the millionaires into 5-cm/2-inch squares. I find it helps to warm the knife up slightly to get a clean cut through the chocolate.

Serve or store in an airtight container for up to 3 days.

rocky road bars

I make these rocky road bars when I make either my campfire pie (page 128) or marshmallows (page 123) as it is a good way of using up the off-cuts and leftovers from both. You can mix up and interchange the ingredients as much as you like, as long as you stick roughly to the same ratio of fillings to chocolate, oil and honey. These are super-indulgent and really hit the spot for my inner chocaholic!

100 g/2½ cups mini marshmallows (or off-cuts from other recipes, see Note)

300 g/10½ oz. dairy-free dark/bittersweet chocolate

50 g/3½ tablespoons coconut oil

30 g/2 tablespoons honey (optional)

1 teaspoon pure vanilla extract

160 g/1⅓ cups mixed pistachios and flaked/slivered almonds, chopped

40 g/¼ cup goji berries (or other organic dried fruit)

a 23-cm/9-inch square deep baking pan lined with baking parchment

MAKES 10–14

Cut the marshmallows into small pieces, roughly 1-cm/⅜-inch square.

Melt together the chocolate, coconut oil, honey and vanilla in a saucepan set over low heat. Stir the ingredients to combine and pour into a large mixing bowl to cool down so that the marshmallows don't melt when added.

Add the pistachios and almonds, goji berries and marshmallows (keep a small handful of nuts and berries back to sprinkle on top for decoration) and mix evenly through the chocolate.

Pour the mixture into the prepared baking pan, sprinkle with the reserved nuts and berries, and put in the fridge to set.

Note: If using off-cuts, you will need to dust the marshmallows lightly with arrowroot before you add them to the mixture so that they aren't too sticky.

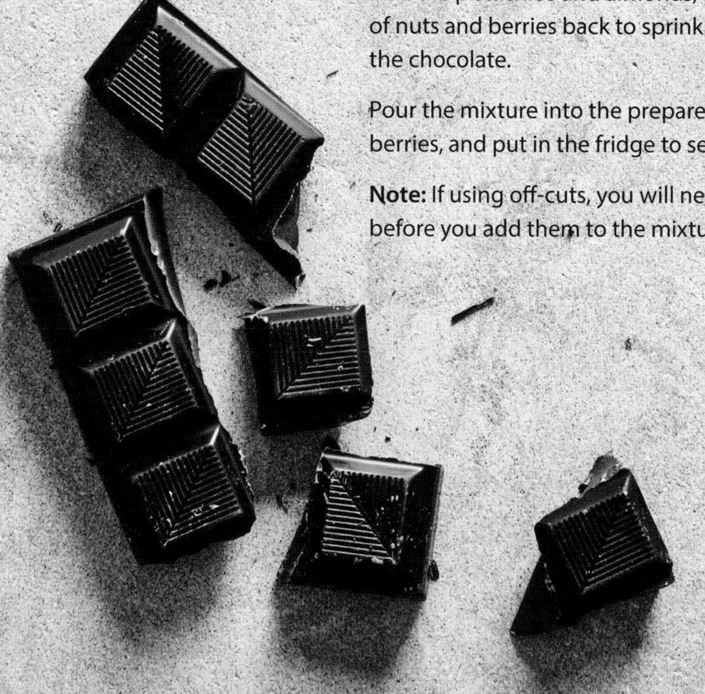

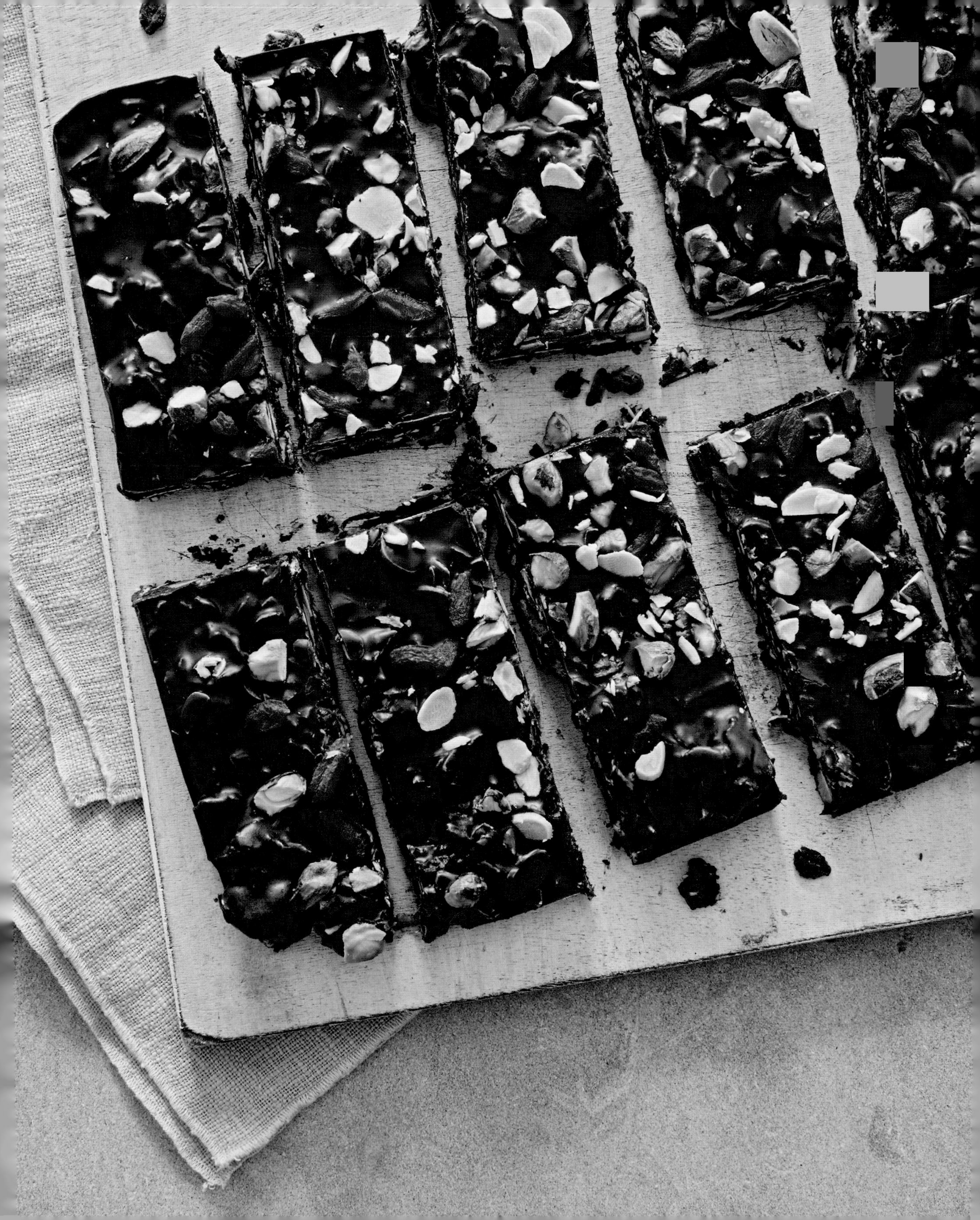

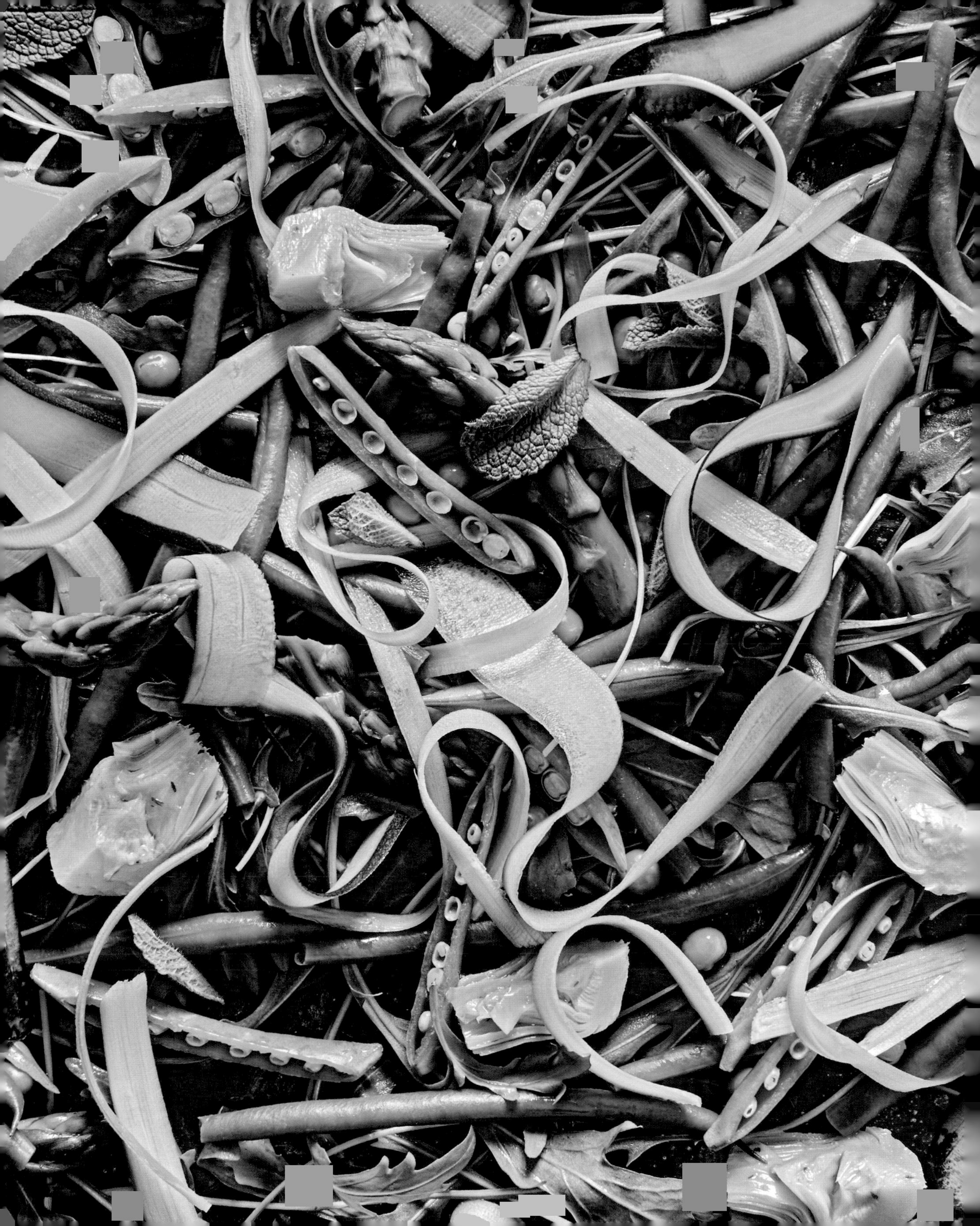

salads, soups and sandwiches

These lighter dishes are perfect for lunch, but also great for an evening meal if you don't fancy anything too heavy. The recipes in this chapter are mostly protein and veg-based, quick and simple, but with a few extra additions to keep things exciting.

squid spaghetti

8–12 baby squid (tentacles included)
a handful of fresh mint leaves, chopped, plus extra to garnish
2 garlic cloves, finely chopped
olive oil, to drizzle
flesh of 1 mango, diced
1/2 fresh chilli/chile, deseeded and finely diced
freshly squeezed juice of 1–2 limes, to taste
a sliver of red onion, thinly sliced (the amount is up to you – I don't think the dish needs much)
1–2 handfuls of seaweed spaghetti (or 3–4 nori sheets)
1–2 carrots, peeled into ribbons
Pickled Carrot and Ginger (optional, page 77), to serve
lime wedges, to serve

SERVES 4

You can make this dish up without the seaweed spaghetti and have it as a salad. I personally really like the spaghetti and I know it's good for me – I buy mine from my local health food shop. Discovering new ingredients is all part of cooking Paleo. Alternatively, replace with spiralized veg.

First prepare the baby squid. Cut rings from half of the squid bodies, then cut the rest in half and score with criss-cross lines. Trim the tentacles and put all the pieces in a large mixing bowl. Sprinkle over the chopped mint and garlic, and drizzle with enough olive oil to coat. Cover and put in the fridge to marinate until ready to serve – you will cook it just before serving.

In a separate bowl, mix together the mango, chilli/chile, lime juice and red onion to make a salsa. Set aside until ready to serve.

The spaghetti is quite strong in flavour and so I don't allow very much per person. If you can't find it then you can also chop up nori sheets and sprinkle the seaweed through the dish to achieve the same flavour. Cook the spaghetti in a saucepan of boiling water for 15 minutes, or as instructed on the packet. Strain and set aside.

Blanch the carrot ribbons in a saucepan of simmering water for just a few seconds to refresh them.

Use the spaghetti and carrots as your base on serving plates. Mix through the mango salsa, then cook the squid.

Preheat a griddle pan over high heat and when very hot add the marinated squid. It will sizzle and turn up at the edges, and cook very quickly in just a couple of minutes.

Add the squid to the serving plates and carefully combine the ingredients but so that the squid and mango stay visible. Sprinkle with a little extra chopped mint and drizzle with a little olive oil. Serve with pickled carrot and ginger (if using) and lime wedges on the side to squeeze over.

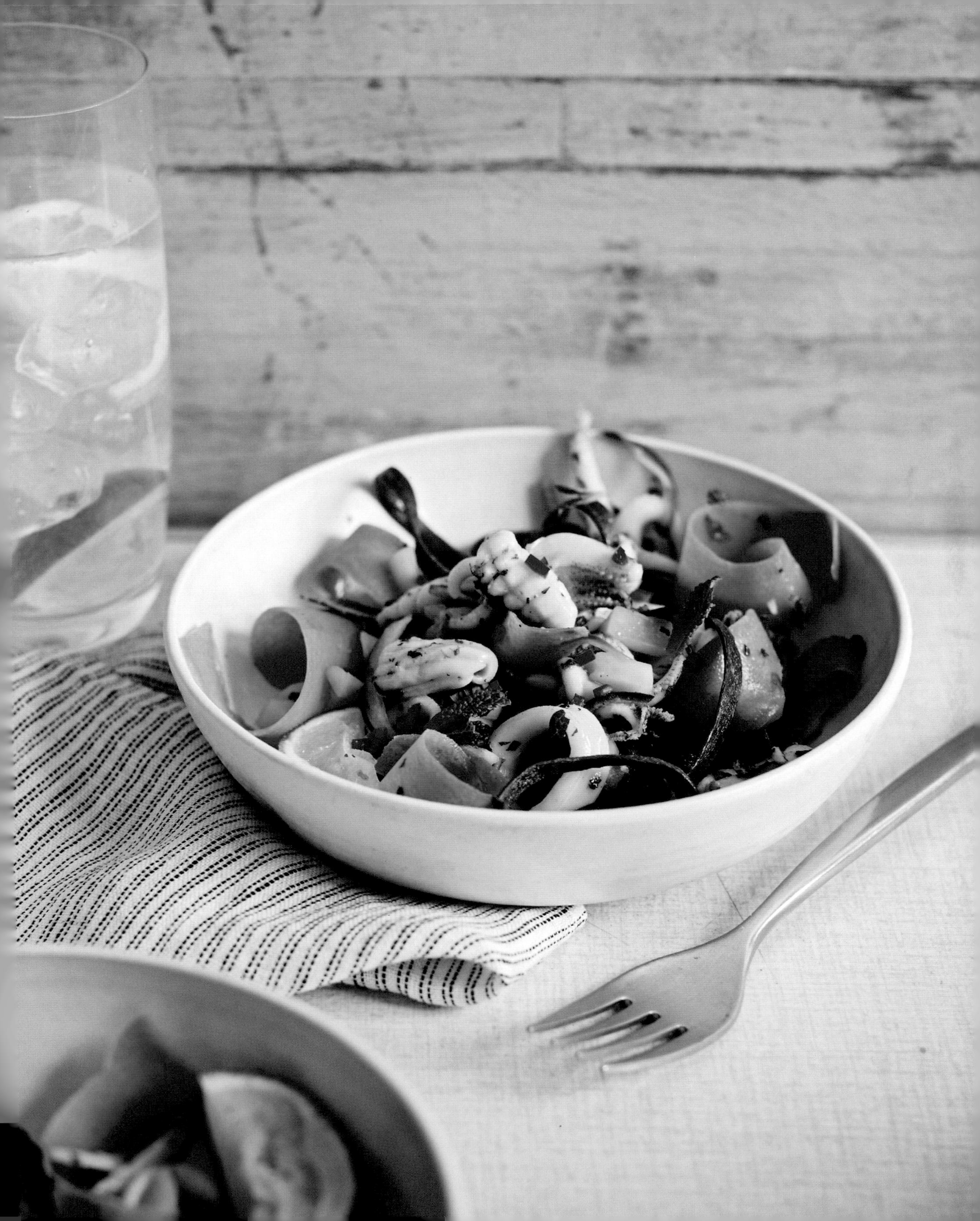

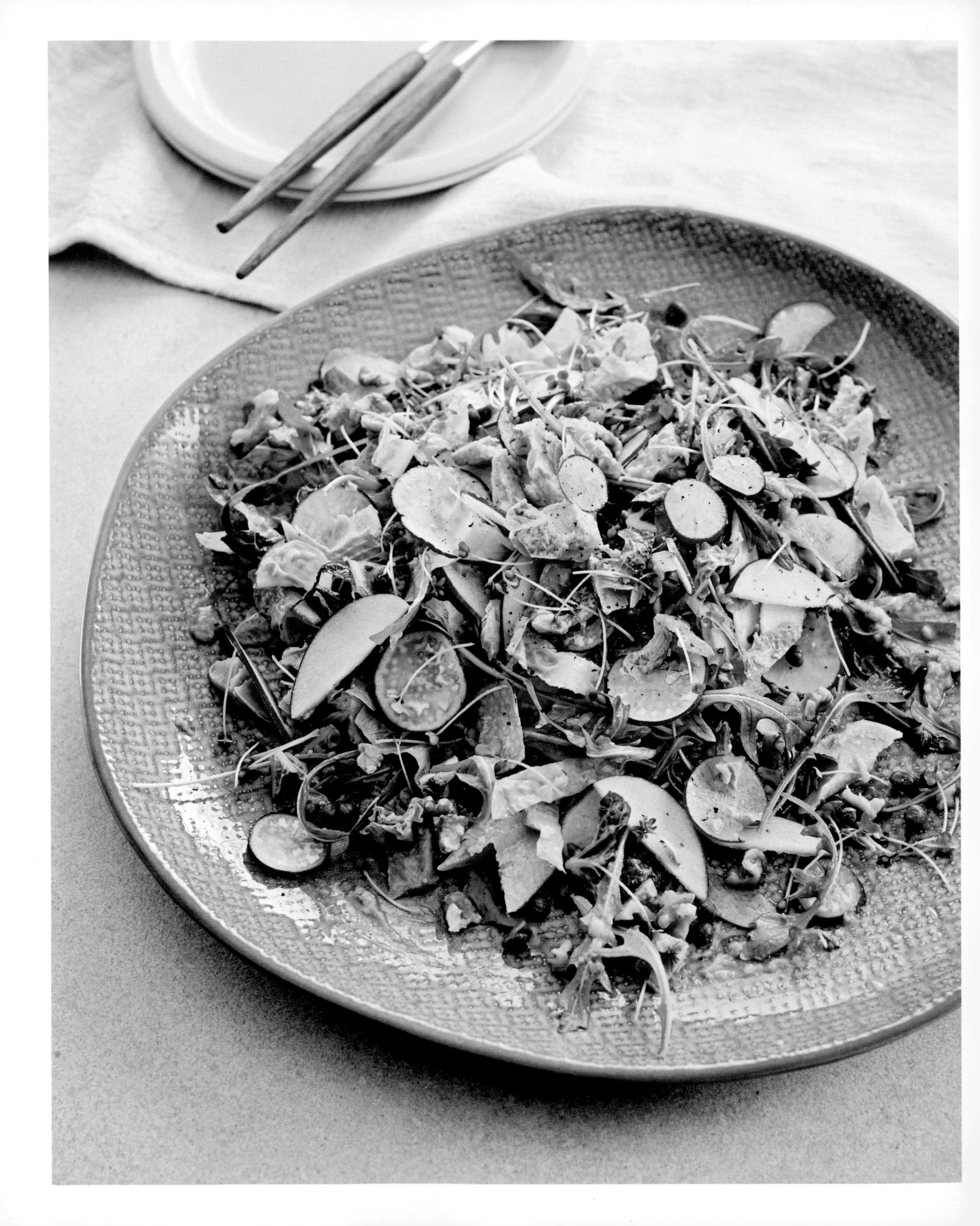

trout salad

A quick, light and easy lunch. Top tip: I like to hold back a few of the fresh ingredients and add them at the very end to keep their colours vibrant and visible. Great for snapping on Instagram to make your friends drool!

½ Pink Lady® apple, thinly sliced

a handful of pink or purple radishes, thinly sliced

½–1 lemon, to squeeze over to taste

1 ripe avocado

a handful of lettuce, shredded

1–2 handfuls of baby rocket/ arugula

a small handful of walnuts (or pecans), roughly chopped

1–2 tablespoons capers

1 tub salad cress

2 fillets good-quality smoked trout

olive oil, to drizzle

black pepper, to season

SERVES 2

Put the sliced apple and radish in a large mixing bowl and squeeze over a little of the lemon juice to stop the apple from discolouring.

In a separate bowl, mash the avocado until smooth, squeeze in the rest of the lemon juice, add the lettuce and rocket/arugula and mix around so that the leaves are nicely 'dressed'.

Scatter the rest of the ingredients into the bowl, including the apple and radish mixture and flake the trout in at the end so that you don't mush it up too much.

Season with a little black pepper, drizzle with olive oil and add an extra little squeeze of lemon if required. Serve immediately.

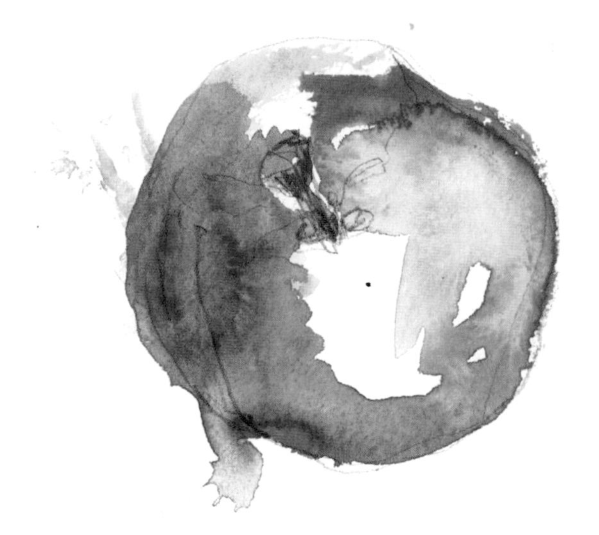

ceviche

Luckily, I live near the south coast of England so can get really fresh, local fish fairly easily. I wouldn't advise making ceviche with anthing but very fresh fish. If you are worried about serving fish that has been 'cooked' in a marinade, then the dressing and salad here is great on top of, or mixed in with, a pan-fried (skin-side down) fillet of sea bass.

2 fillets sea bass

freshly squeezed juice of 2 oranges

3 sweet baby (bell) peppers (if possible, use red, yellow and orange to add colour)

2 baby fennel (leaves on), shredded

2 shallots, thinly sliced

a handful of fresh flat-leaf parsley (stalks and all), finely chopped

a small handful of shredded chicory leaves

salt and pink or black pepper, to season

to serve

salad cress

olive oil, to drizzle

½ lime, to squeeze over

SERVES 2

Prepare the fish by removing the skin and chopping into 2.5-cm/1-inch pieces. Put in a large mixing bowl, cover with clingfilm/plastic wrap and put in the fridge until ready to serve.

Mix together the orange juice, baby (bell) peppers, fennel, shallots and parsley. Season with salt and pepper (I prefer pink pepper in this dish), cover and put in the fridge until ready to serve.

Immediately before serving, mix together the fish into the orange mixture. Stir through the chicory and plate. Top with salad cress, drizzle with olive oil and squeeze over the lime juice. Enjoy!

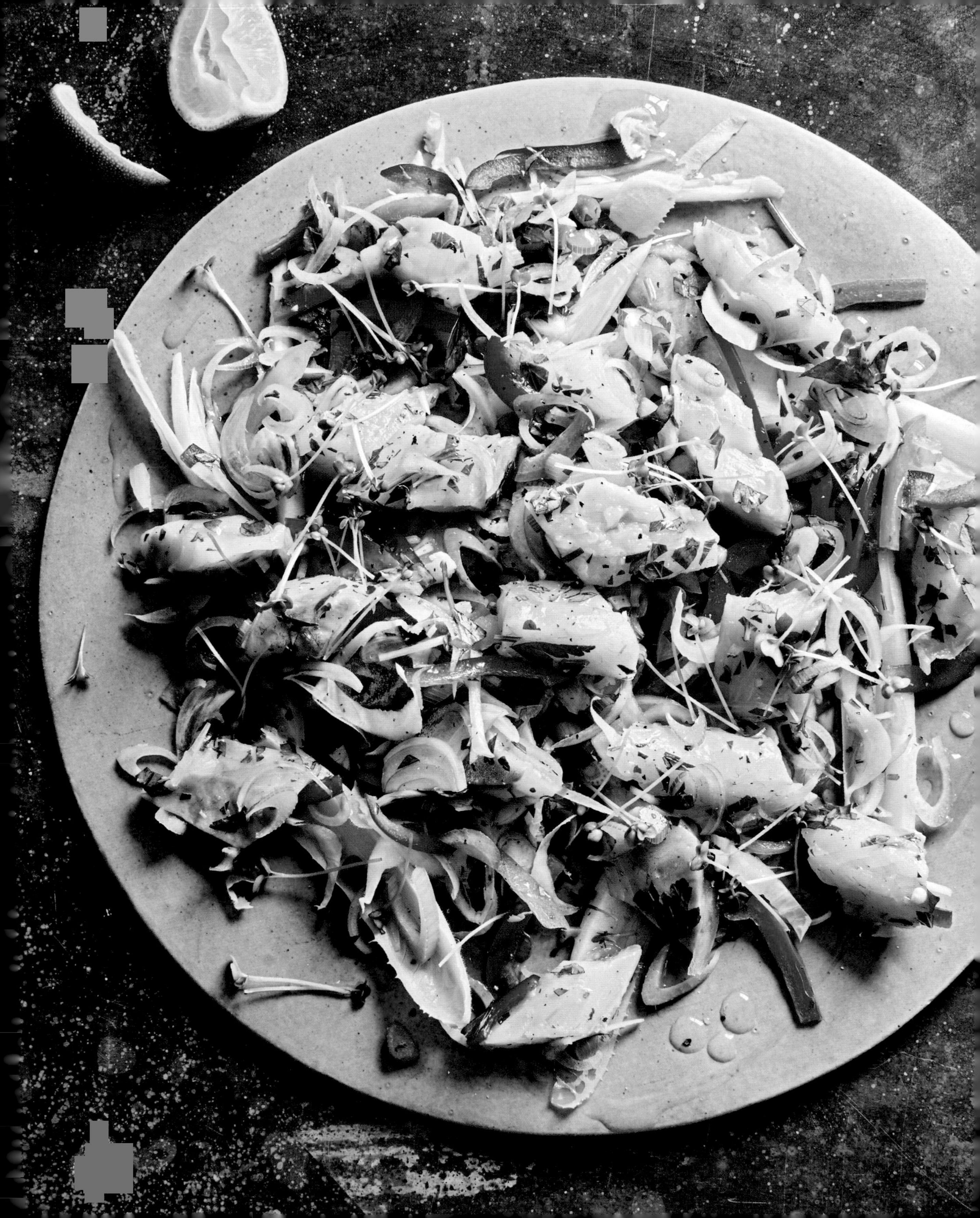

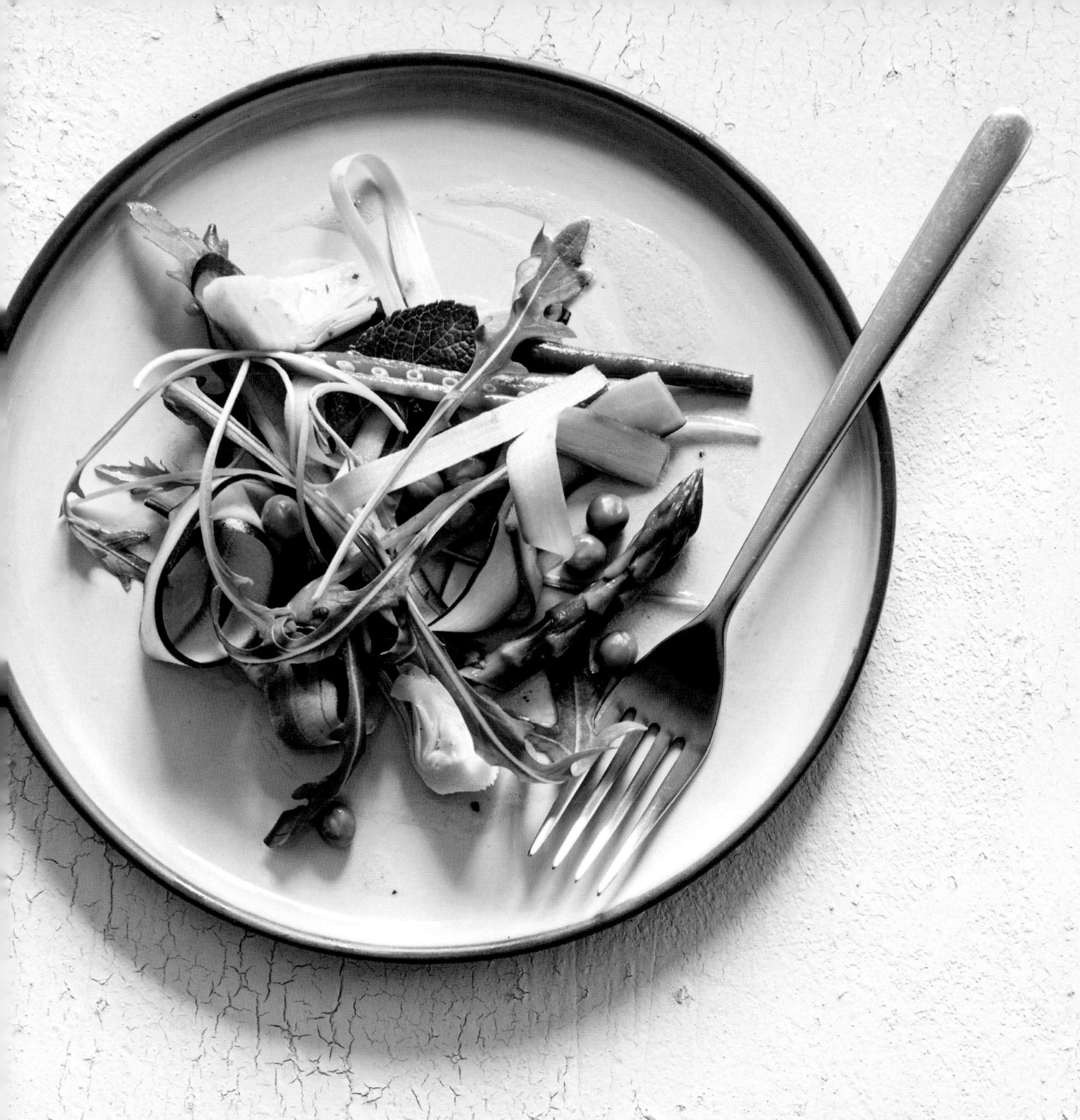

Salads are the quickest, easiest, freshest way to get loads of green into your diet! Enjoy them as the main event for a garden picnic or alongside a host of barbecue foods on beautiful summer days.

summer green salad

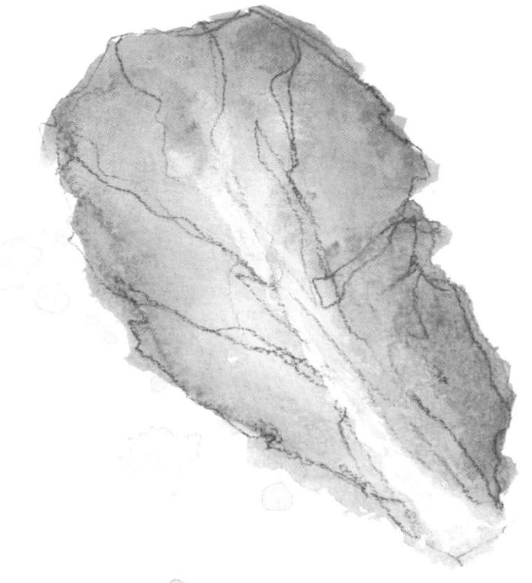

a bunch of asparagus

a handful of green/French beans

a handful of sugar snap peas (or mangetout/snow peas)

a handful of freshly shelled peas

$^{1}/_{2}$ courgette/zucchini

a 180-g/6$^{1}/_{2}$-oz. jar of artichoke hearts in olive oil, drained

a handful of rocket/arugula

a handful of fresh mint leaves, chopped

salt and black pepper, to season

dressing

1 teaspoon Dijon mustard

freshly squeezed juice of $^{1}/_{2}$–1 lemon, to taste

olive oil, to drizzle

a baking sheet lined with baking parchment

SERVES 4

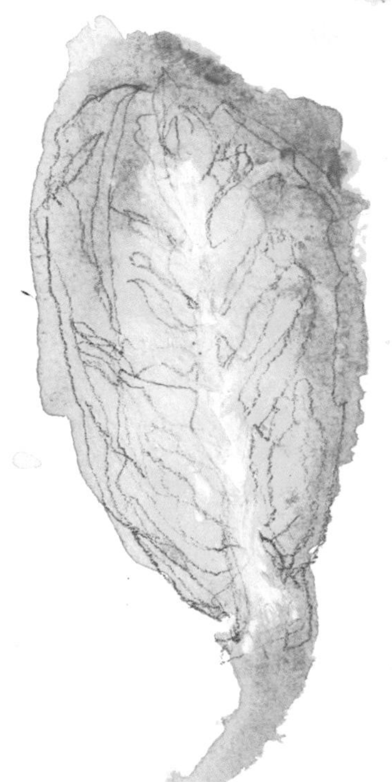

Blanch the asparagus, beans, sugar snap peas and fresh peas in a saucepan of simmering water for 1–2 minutes, then strain and plunge immediately into a bowl filled with iced water to suspend the cooking. You may need to do this is batches.

Use a speed peeler to peel lengths of the courgette/zucchini and cooked asparagus, keeping the asparagus tops in tact.

To make the dressing, mix together the mustard with the lemon juice then drizzle in some olive oil and taste. Alter the quantities to your taste and set aside.

Mix all the salad ingredients together, season with salt and pepper and pour over the dressing. Toss to coat, add a little more olive oil if necessary and serve.

tomato and romano pepper soup with vegan rolls

You just can't beat homemade soup. By making it from scratch you can avoid any artificial nasties and let the flavours of the main ingredients sing for themselves accompanied by a great alternative to bread for a Paleo vegan option.

4 garlic cloves

3 red Romano peppers, stalk and seeds removed

800 g/1 3/4 lb. tomatoes

1 1/2 white onions, diced

leaves from 5 sprigs of fresh thyme

a big handful of fresh basil

300 g/10 1/2 oz. celeriac, peeled and roughly chopped

900 ml/1 quart Vegetable Stock (page 17)

salt and black pepper, to season

coconut oil, for frying

good-quality cold-pressed olive oil, to drizzle

vegan rolls

100 g/scant 1 cup milled flaxseeds, plus extra to sprinkle (see Notes)

50 g/1/3 cup tapioca flour

90 g/2/3 cup coconut flour

40 g/1 1/2 oz. psyllium husk

1 teaspoon baking powder

50 g/3 1/2 tablespoons flax egg (see Notes)

a pinch of sea salt flakes

2 tablespoons olive oil

mixed dried herbs

a baking sheet lined with oiled baking parchment

SERVES 4

Preheat the oven to 220°C (425°F) Gas 7.

To make the vegan rolls, mix together the dry ingredients but not the salt in a large mixing bowl. Add the flax egg, salt and 220 ml/scant 1 cup luke-warm water. Mix together quickly and if the dough seems too dry add a little more water. The dry ingredients absorb liquid quickly so try to work fast rather than add too much water.

Roll the dough into four equal balls, brush with the olive oil, sprinkle with a few extra flaxseeds and a little salt. Arrange on the prepared baking sheet.

Bake in the preheated oven for 10 minutes, then turn heat down to 180°C (350°F) Gas 4 and continue to bake for 25 minutes.

Meanwhile, lay the garlic cloves, peeled but still whole, on a baking sheet with the peppers and tomatoes. Roast in the oven at the same time as the rolls for 15–20 minutes.

Put a little coconut oil into a large saucepan, add the onion, thyme and basil. Set over medium heat, then add the celeriac and sauté for 5 minutes or so, until lightly coloured.

Add the roasted vegetables and the stock to the pan, cover with a lid and simmer for about 20 minutes, until the celeriac is soft. Remove the pan from the heat and blend the ingredients together with a handheld electric blender.

Season with salt and pepper, drizzle with olive oil and serve with the vegan rolls.

Notes:

- Flaxseeds/linseeds can be milled at home if you can't get hold of packaged milled flaxseeds/linseeds.
- To make a flax egg, mix 2 tablespoons of the flaxseeds/linseeds with 250 ml/ 1 cup of water in a small saucepan and bring to a gentle simmer over low heat until it becomes like an egg white consistency.
- The rolls can be made in advance and can be stored in an airtight container for up to 3 days.

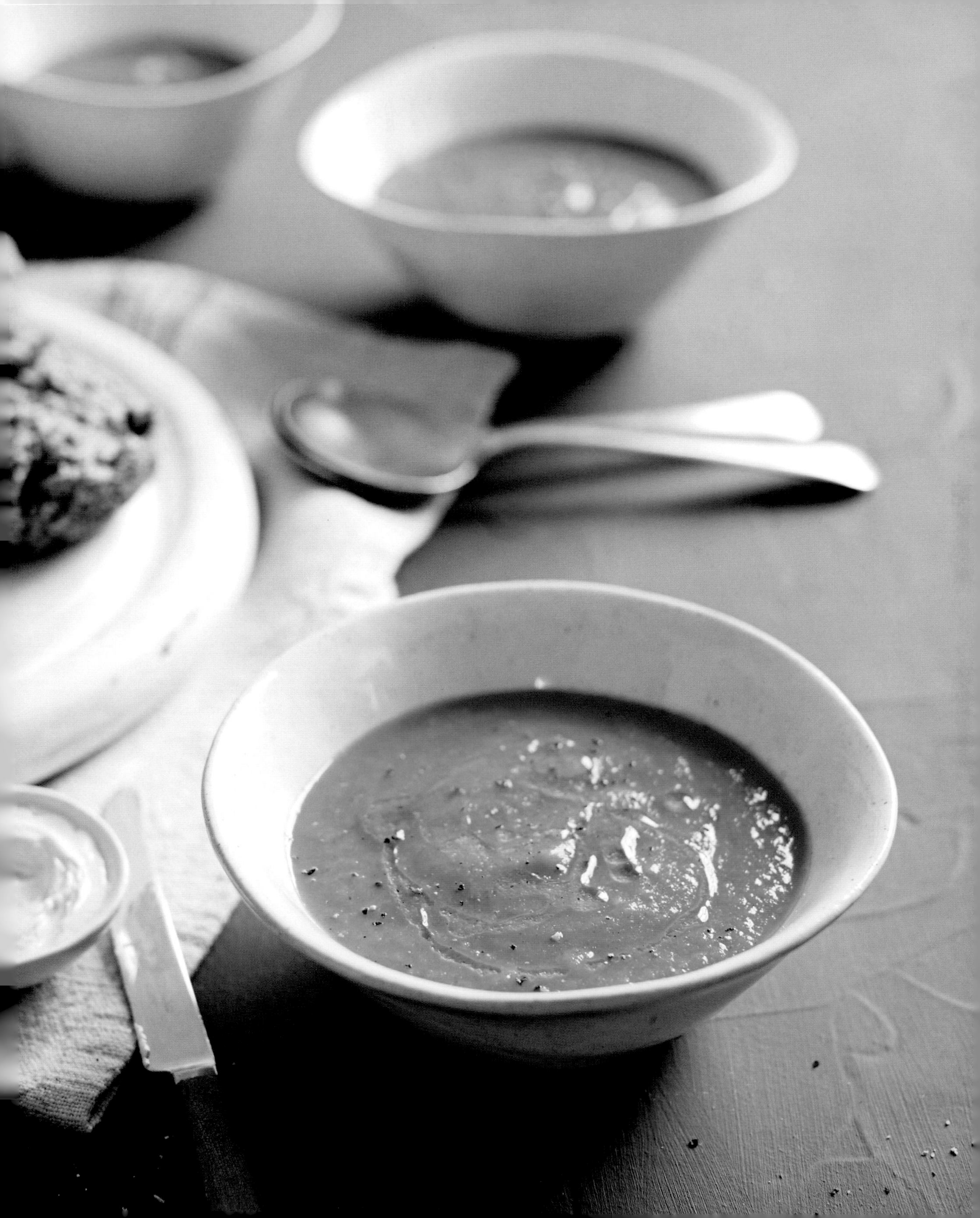

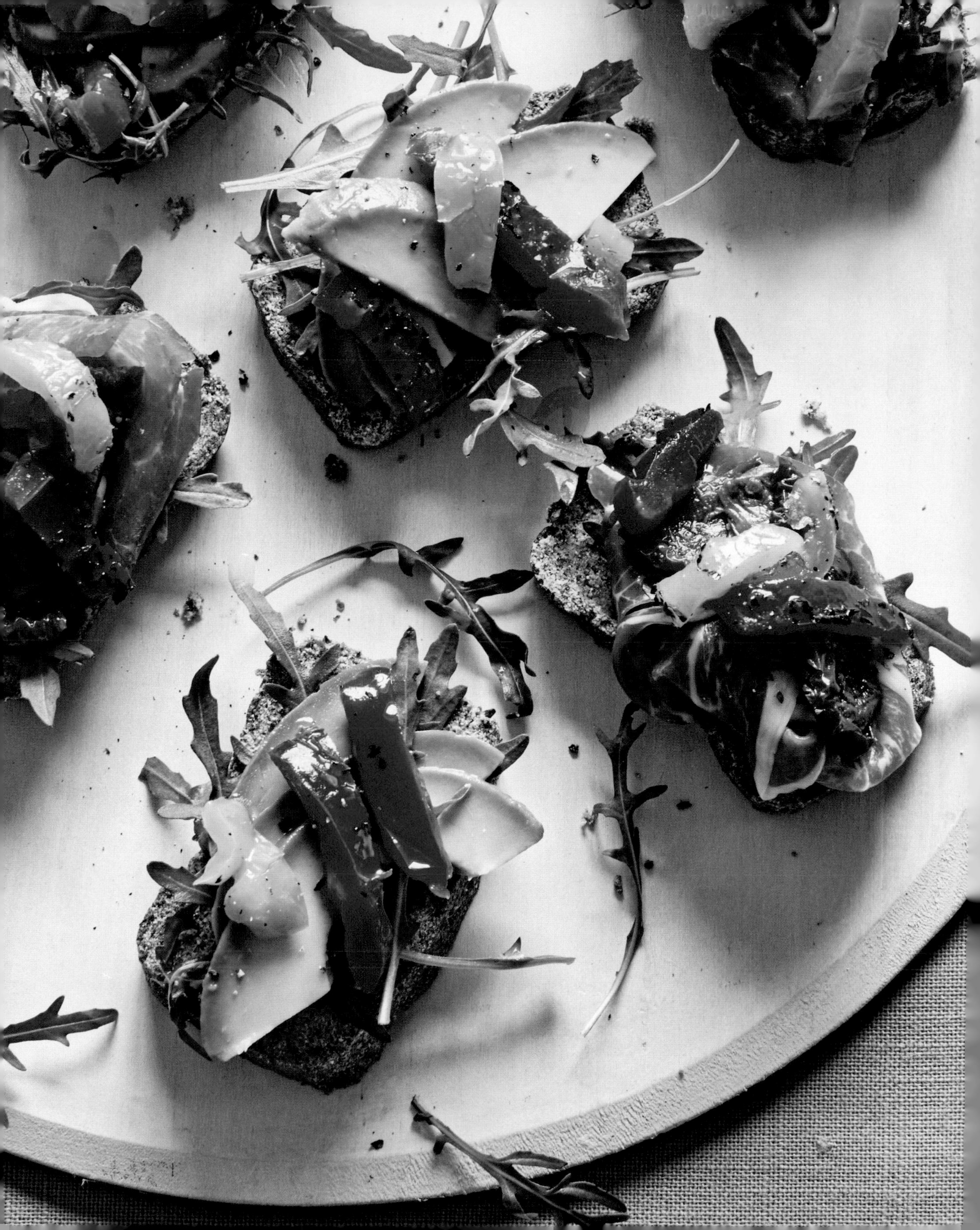

nut-free open sandwiches

Open sandwiches are the best! You can top them with anything you might have knocking around and they are great for using up leftovers to create a quick and easy lunch. I make the bread for these sandwiches in a small loaf pan as it is best served when fresh. It's such an easy bake that you can make it again without too much hassle if you need to. Bear in mind that psyllium husk is very high in fibre and gets your bowel moving so don't have too many slices in one day.

140 g/5 oz. rocket/arugula
flesh of 1 avocado, sliced
4–6 slices Parma ham
a 460-g/16-oz. jar roast (bell) peppers (or home-roasted)
a 280-g/10-oz. jar sun-dried tomatoes (or home-dried)
olive oil, to drizzle
salt and black pepper, to season

nut-free loaf
35 g/¼ cup milled flaxseeds/ linseeds (milled at home if preferred)
50 g/1 cup coconut flour
40 g/¼ cup psyllium husk
1 teaspoon baking powder
a good pinch of sea salt flakes
4 tablespoons olive oil
1 egg plus 1 egg white

a 450-g/1-lb. loaf pan lined with oiled baking parchment

SERVES 4–6

First, make the nut-free loaf. Preheat the oven to 180°C (350°F) Gas 4.

Mix together all the dry ingredients in a large mixing bowl.

In a separate bowl, whisk together the oil, egg and egg white with 175 ml/ ¾ cup of warm water.

Make a well in the centre of the dry ingredients and pour in the wet mixture. Stir together quickly. The coconut flour and the psyllium husk absorb the liquid faster than you would think so be sure to move quickly from the minute you add the egg mixture to when you put the loaf in the oven.

Use your hands to press the mixed 'dough' into the prepared loaf pan.

Bake in the preheated oven for 40 minutes.

Remove from the oven, turn out the loaf from the pan and remove the baking parchment. Cool on a wire rack. Thinly slice the loaf into 8–12 slices.

Put a small heap of rocket/arugula leaves on each slice and top with sliced avocado or Parma ham, then roast (bell) peppers and sun-dried tomatoes. Drizzle with a little olive oil and season with salt and pepper.

Note: Try topping the slices with smoked mackerel mixed with a little good-quality or homemade mayonnaise (page 14) and thin ribbons of cucumber lightly pickled in white wine vinegar. Or to use up any cuts of leftover roast beef, layer up rare beef slices with parsnip remoulade (page 99).

honey and mustard chicken wrap

You can readily buy Paleo wraps made from coconut flour in health food stores or online. So if you haven't got the time to whip up a batch of these flat breads, you can substitute them for store-bought ones. Or, if you don't fancy the wrap, the filling makes a great salad. You could also make the vegan rolls on page 70 and fill them with the chicken for a satisfying chicken burger.

2 heaped tablespoons honey
2 heaped tablespoons wholegrain mustard
2 chicken breasts, cooked and shredded
4 shallots, thinly sliced
1 onion, thinly sliced
leaves of 5 fresh thyme sprigs, chopped
a drizzle of olive oil
a dash of red wine vinegar

Paleo flat breads

160 g/scant 2 cups almond flour
240 g/2 cups arrowroot
a pinch of salt
2 tablespoons olive oil

to serve

mayonnaise
shredded lettuce

SERVES 2–4

Begin by making the Paleo flat breads. Mix together the almond flour, arrowroot and salt in a large mixing bowl. Make a well in the centre then add the oil and 140 ml/scant 2/3 cup of water. Mix well and bring together into a ball. The dough should be easy to handle without being too sticky.

Pull the dough into four equal parts and roll each part into a ball. Using an oiled rolling pin, roll each ball out relatively thin onto a lightly floured piece of baking parchment – you may need a little extra arrowroot to stop it from sticking.

Set a non-stick frying pan/skillet over medium heat and brush with a little oil. The pan needs to be almost dry, so don't get carried away with the oil.

Using the baking parchment to lift the flat breads to the pan, cook on each side and keep warm until ready to serve, or cool and freeze immediately if not serving right away. (The flat breads can be defrosted and warmed in a dry pan.)

Preheat the oven to 180°C (350°F) Gas 4.

For the filling, warm the honey and wholegrain mustard in a saucepan over low heat. Once combined, remove 1 tablespoon and reserve before adding the shredded chicken.

Put the shallots, onion, thyme leaves, olive oil, red wine vinegar and reserved honey and mustard in a separate saucepan and cook over low heat until the shallots and onion start to crisp slightly and become caramelized. The sauce should reduce down. Transfer the honey and mustard chicken and the caramelized shallots and onion to a baking dish and put in the preheated oven for 10 minutes to warm through.

Spread some mayo on the flat breads and add some shredded lettuce, top with chicken and shallots, wrap up and enjoy!

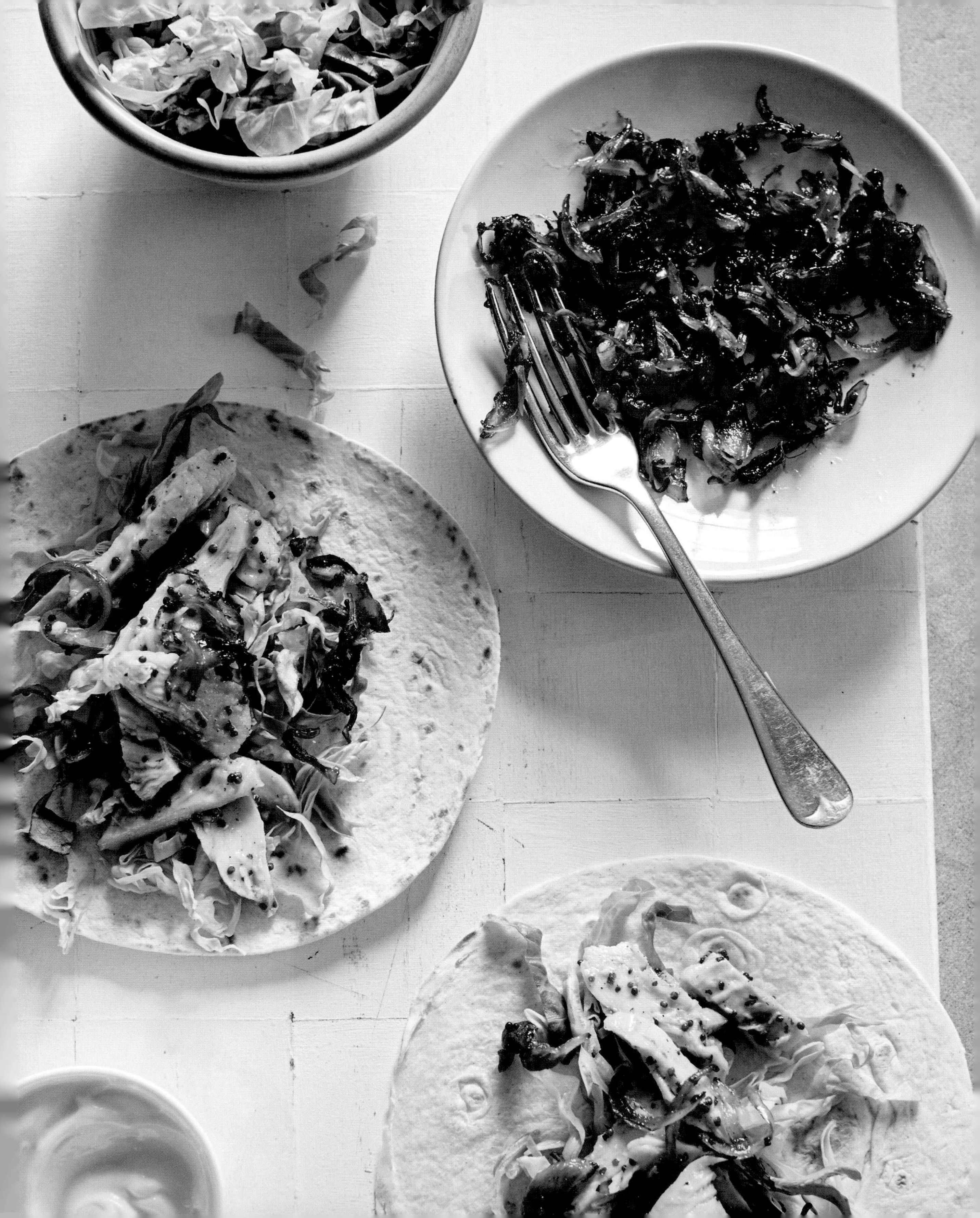

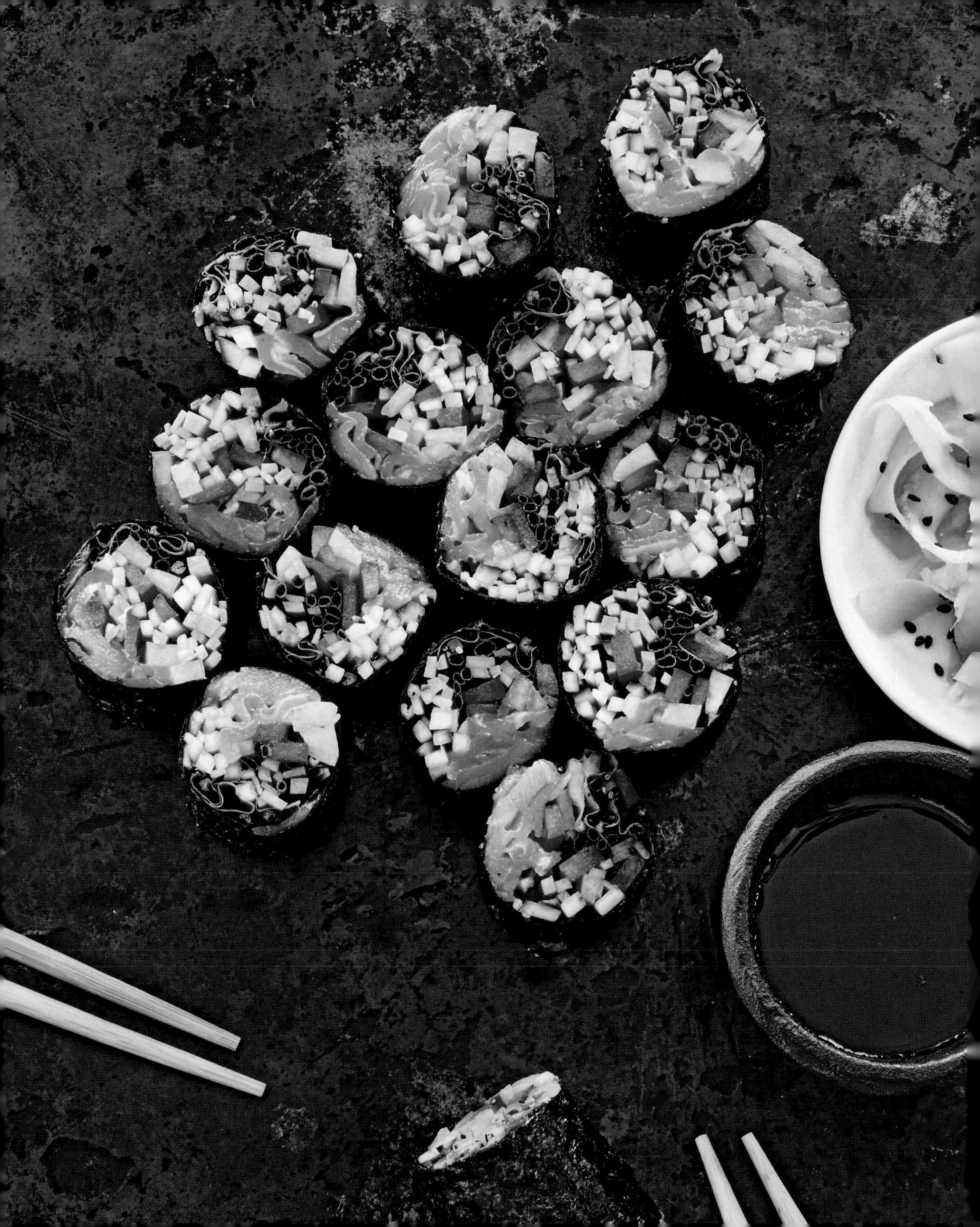

nori rolls with pickled carrot and ginger

This dish is super-healthy. It is easy to make and perfect for a quick lunch or appetizer. Once you've got the hang of rolling the ingredients up, try adding your own fillings.

1 carrot, very thinly sliced into strips
1/3 cucumber (deseeded), very thinly sliced into strips
1/2 red (bell) pepper, very thinly sliced into strips
4 nori sheets
200 g/7 oz. smoked salmon, roughly chopped
a bunch each of fresh chives and fresh coriander/cilantro
a handful of baby leaf rocket/arugula

pickled carrot and ginger
1 lemongrass stalk
2 star anise
100 ml/1/3 cup white wine vinegar
1 tablespoon salt
1 tablespoon pure maple syrup
4 carrots, cut into ribbons
a 7.5-cm/3-inch piece of fresh ginger, peeled and cut into ribbons

to serve
sesame oil
black sesame seeds
liquid coconut aminos

a 300-ml/10-fl. oz. capacity sterilized glass jar with an airtight lid

MAKES 20

First prepare the pickled carrot and ginger. Put all of the ingredients except the carrot and ginger in a saucepan. Pour over 120 ml/1/2 cup of water and warm over low–medium heat. Put the carrot and ginger ribbons in a sterilized glass jar and pour over the warmed vinaigrette. Screw the lid on tightly, turn upside down while still warm and leave to cool completely. The heat and gravity will create a seal in the jar. The pickle will be ready to use after a couple of hours. Store in the fridge for up to 1 week.

Take a few pieces of ginger from the pickled carrot and ginger pot and very thinly slice into strips. Set aside with the other sliced vegetables ready to roll.

Lay out the nori sheets. Put a strip of salmon horizontally across the middle, then add a few lengths of chive, coriander/cilantro (stalks and all), the sliced vegetables and ginger and top with a little rocket/arugula.

Drizzle with sesame oil and sprinkle with sesame seeds. Then, when you are ready to roll, slightly dampen the nori sheet with the pickling juice from the pickled carrot and ginger by dipping your fingers into the jar and just dabbing across the sheet. Roll up tightly, cut each roll into 5 equal parts and arrange on a serving platter.

Serve with pickled carrot and ginger and liquid coconut aminos to dip into.

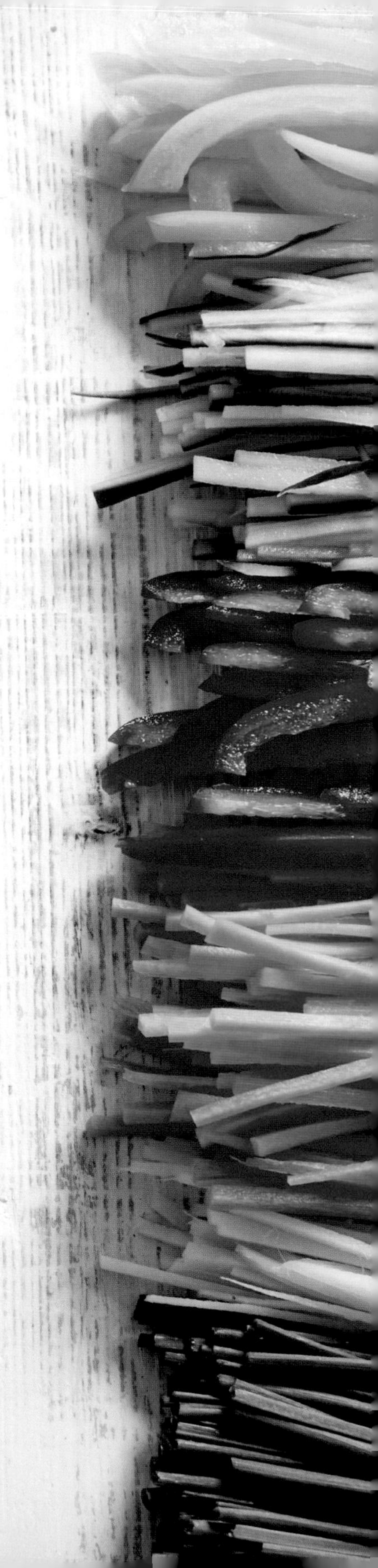

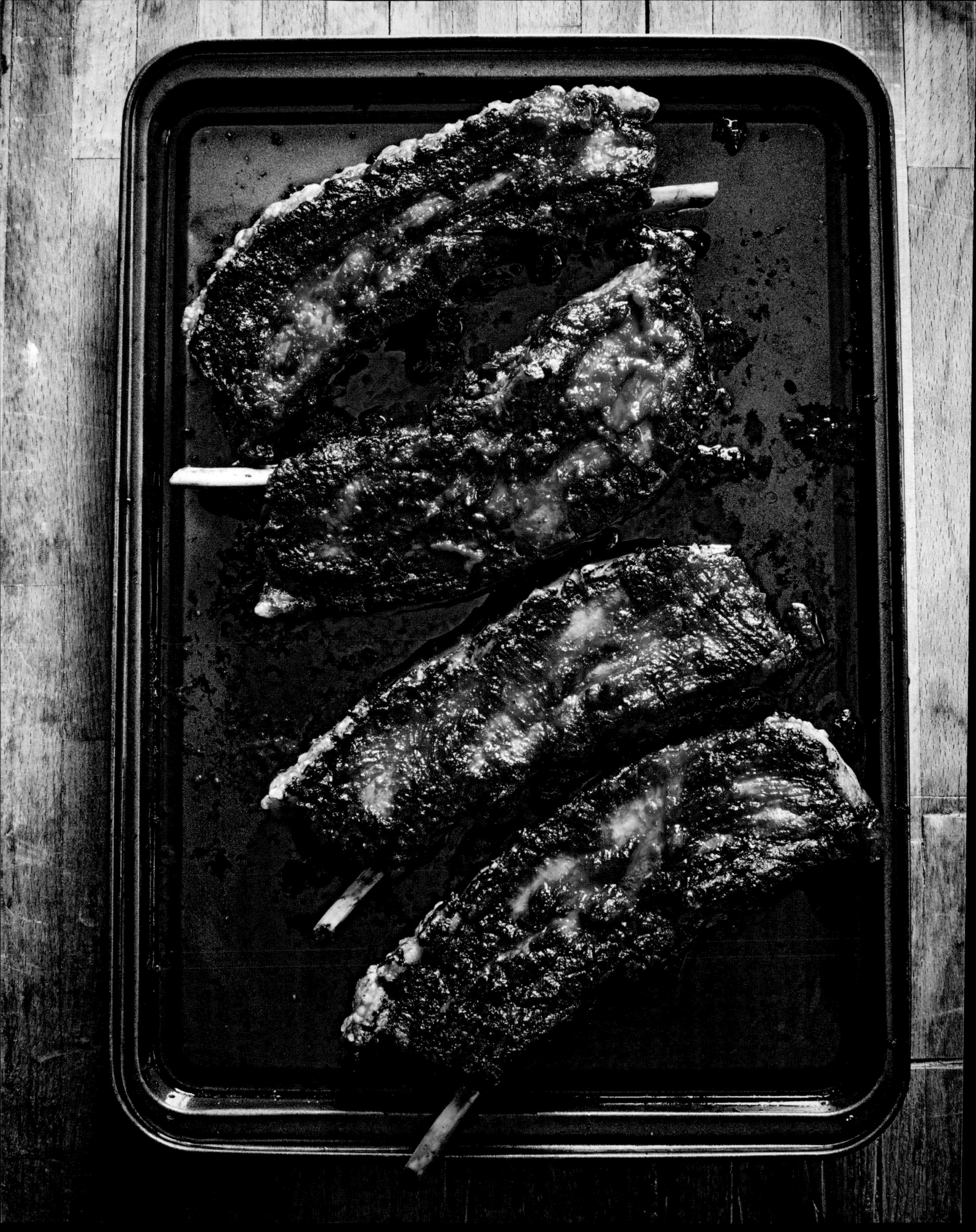

main meals

I like to think of my main meal of the day as my time to refuel – it's important to load up on nutritionally dense food to keep your body happy. But it is also when I like to host and entertain. To me, there is nothing better than sharing food with friends and family, it's in my nature and I love it.

sweet potato gnocchi with fried eggs

500 g/18 oz. sweet potato (skin on)

130 g/1$^1/_3$ cups almond flour, plus extra for rolling out

65 g/$^1/_2$ cup arrowroot

65 g/$^1/_2$ cup coconut flour

1 egg, lightly whisked

4 eggs

olive oil, for frying

salt and black pepper, to season

tomato sauce

3 heaped tablespoons coconut butter

zest of $^1/_2$–1 lemon, to taste

freshly squeezed juice of 1–2 lemons, to taste

4 tablespoons chopped fresh or dried sage

4 celery stalks/ribs, finely diced

400 g/14 oz. cherry or large tomatoes, finely diced

a few big handfuls of spinach

SERVES 4

A great alternative to pasta – I hadn't actually eaten gnocchi before writing this recipe, but after trying it out I thought it added something new and exciting to my Paleo repertoire.

To make the gnocchi, cook the sweet potato as a whole potato with the skin left on. Either boil for 10 minutes or until soft and cooked through – leaving the skin on means that the potato won't absorb too much liquid – or roast in an oven at 180°C (350°F) Gas 4 for 45 minutes–1 hour. Once the potato is cooked, peel and set on paper towels to absorb any excess water. It doesn't need to be bone dry, you just don't want to add too much excess moisture to the mixture.

Put the almond flour, arrowroot and coconut flour in a bowl and mix well.

Mash the sweet potato with a fork or beat with a spoon to make it smooth. Spoon onto a clean surface or sheet of baking parchment. Spread it out so it has a well in the middle. Sprinkle about half of the flour mixture and a pinch of salt on top and pour the whisked egg in the middle. I add the flour in stages as I find you might not need all of it depending on the moisture from your potato. Paleo flours absorb moisture much more easily than other flours so it depends how much excess moisture there is. Knead the ingredients together with your hands until a dough is formed. Add more of the flour mixture if required but be careful not to over-work the dough.

Pull off small bits of dough, roughly 10 g/$^1/_2$ oz. each and roll into balls. Lightly press down with the back of a fork to flattened slightly and mark with lines.

Put the coconut butter, lemon zest and juice, sage, celery and tomatoes in a frying pan/skillet and set over medium heat. Sauté for a few minutes to soften the celery and break down the tomatoes.

Bring a saucepan of water to the boil, then add the gnocchi. You might need to do this in 2–3 batches depending on the size of your saucepan. Cook for 2–3 minutes and remove the gnocchi from the pan with a slotted spoon when they rise to the surface.

In a separate frying pan/skillet, fry the eggs in a little olive oil so that the white is cooked and the yolk still runny.

Transfer the cooked gnocchi into the pan with the celery and tomatoes and stir to coat. Add the spinach and cook for another couple of minutes.

Season with salt, pepper and lemon juice and spoon onto serving plates or bowls. Top each one with a fried egg and serve.

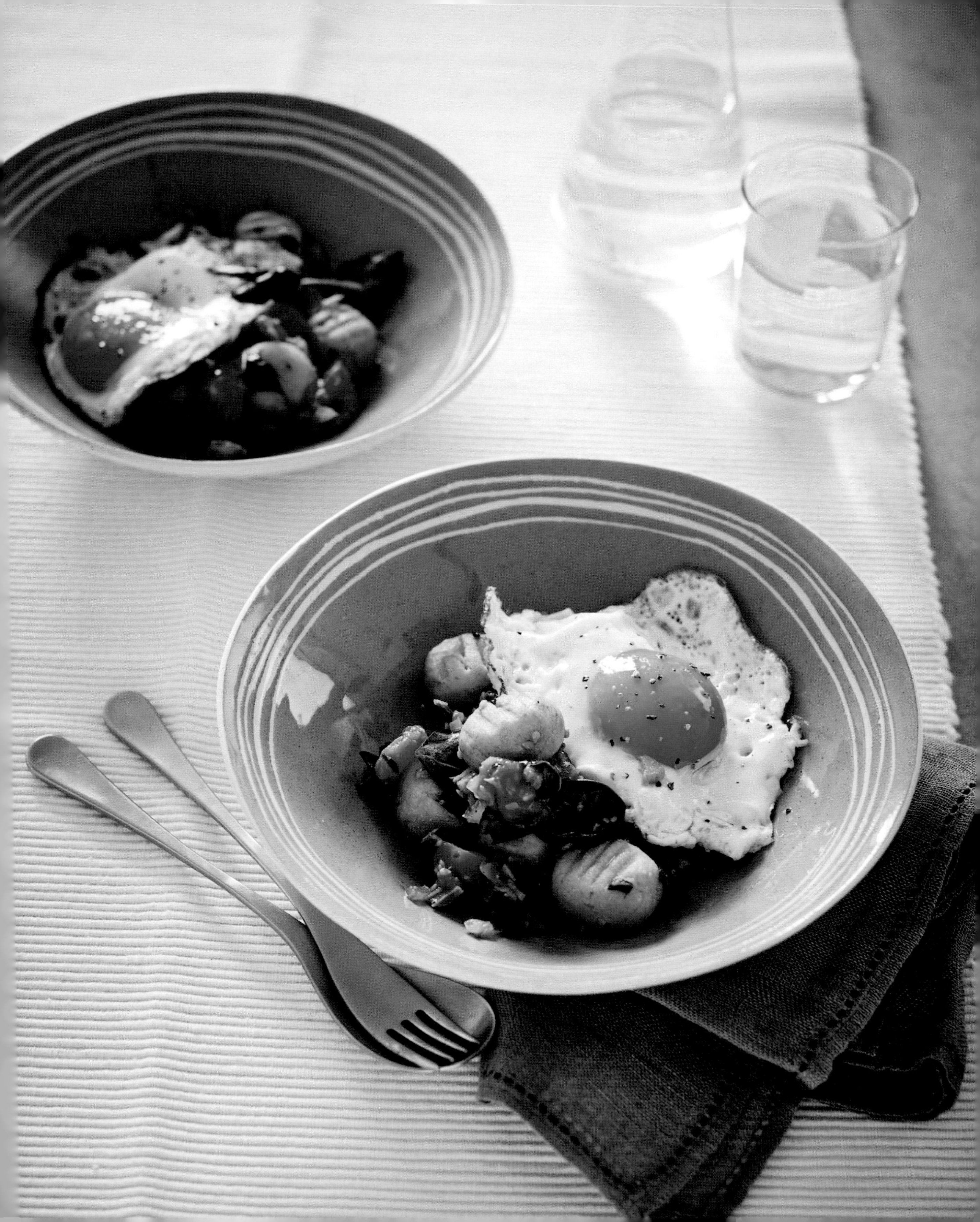

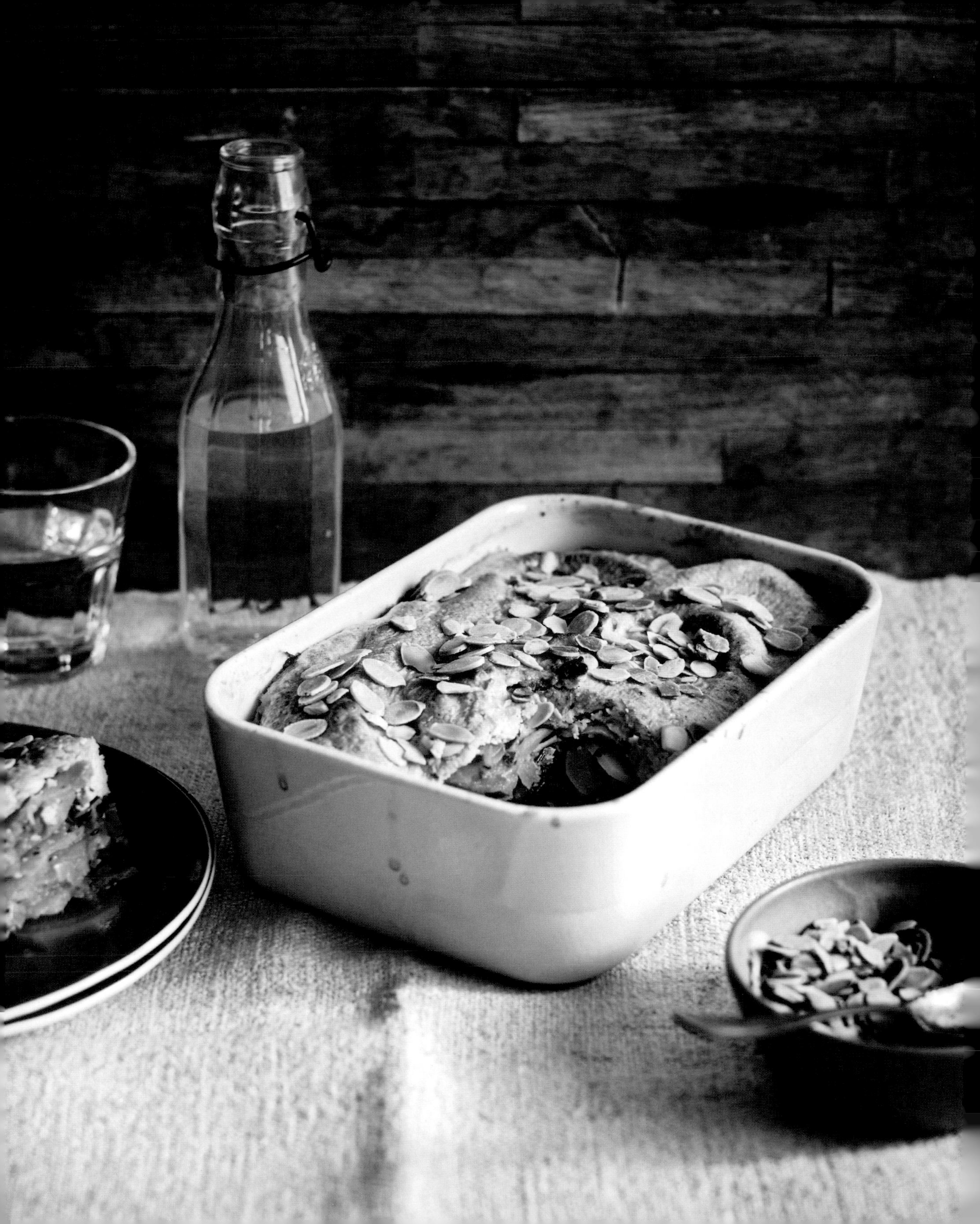

winter root vegetable gratin

1 tablespoon coconut butter

1 heaped tablespoon each of chopped fresh parsley and rosemary

leaves of 8 sprigs fresh thyme

2 bay leaves

2 celery stalks/ribs, finely diced

1 onion, finely diced

4–5 ladles Vegetable Stock (page 17)

250 g/9 oz. white turnip, thinly sliced

250 g/9 oz. swede/rutabaga, peeled and thinly sliced

250 g/9 oz. butternut squash, peeled and thinly sliced

black pepper, to season

toasted flaked/slivered almonds, to serve

topping

200 g/1 3/4 cup cashews, soaked in water

1/2 teaspoon salt

freshly squeezed juice of 1/2 lemon

1/2 teaspoon mixed dried herbs (I use a dried Italian herb mix)

a 1-litre/quart capacity casserole dish, greased with coconut butter

a high-powered blender (I use a NutriBullet)

SERVES 4–6

This is quite a hearty vegan meal, which is warming enough to serve straight from the pan and I actually really enjoy it served on its own or with some simple sauteéd or steamed green veg on the side.

Preheat the oven to 180°C (350°F) Gas 4.

Put the coconut butter in a large saucepan over medium heat. Add the herbs, celery and onion, and sauté for a few minutes. Pour over the stock and cook for a little while longer.

Layer the sliced root veg in the prepared casserole dish – I tend to mix and match the vegetables in a layer – and, between each layer, add a layer of the cooked onions and celery, removing the bay leaves. Pile the layers up high as the casserole shrinks as it cooks, season with black pepper and pour over the remaining stock – you may not need all the stock but there should be enough to steam through the veg, bearing in mind that it will evaporate during cooking.

Put the dish on top of a baking sheet in case of spillages and bake in the preheated oven for 45 minutes, or until the veg is cooked.

To make the topping, blend all the ingredients in a high-powered blender with 6 tablespoons of water. The mixture should be smooth. If it seems too thick add a little more water. It should have the consistency of a creamy white sauce or béchamel.

Remove the casserole dish from the oven and spread the topping over the cooked vegetables. Return to the oven and bake for another 10 minutes, or until golden.

Sprinkle with almonds immediately before serving.

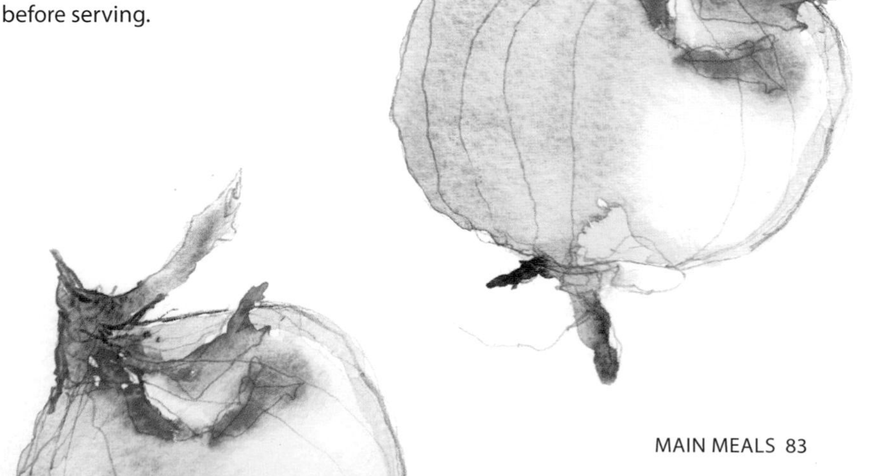

pizza sauce
1 red (bell) pepper, chopped
5 medium tomatoes, halved
3 garlic cloves
1/2 tablespoon dried oregano

pizza base
80 g/1/2 cup arrowroot
130 g/1 cup tapioca flour
190 g/2 cups ground almonds
1 tablespoon mixed dried herbs (or dried oregano)
1 garlic clove
salt and black pepper, to season

tapenade
70 g/3/4 cup pitted/stoned black olives
70 g/3/4 cup pitted/stoned green olives
1–2 tablespoons capers, squeezed of excess liquid
juice of 1/2 lemon
2 big handfuls of fresh basil
70 ml/5 tablespoons extra virgin olive oil

toppings
1 cooked chicken breast, sliced
a small handful of sun-dried tomatoes, chopped
1/4–1/2 green or yellow courgette/zucchini, shaved
a handful of rocket/arugula
fresh basil leaves, torn
1 teaspoon dried oregano

2 baking sheets lined with baking parchment, 1 brushed with olive oil

a high-powered blender (I use a NutriBullet)

pizza stone (optional)

MAKES 1 30-CM/ 12-INCH PIZZA

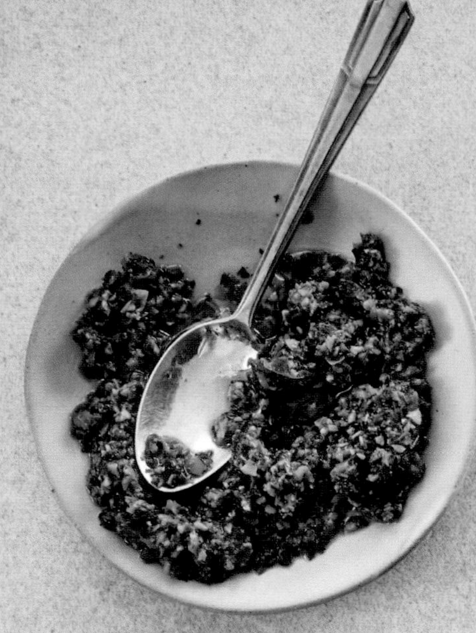

paleo pizza

A healthy pizza base with good carbs and protein from a mixture of flours and almonds.

Begin by preparing the sauce. Preheat the oven to 180°C (350°F) Gas 4.

Put the red (bell) pepper, tomatoes and garlic on the prepared baking sheet without oil, sprinkle with the oregano and season with salt and pepper. Bake in the preheated oven for 20 minutes. Remove the roast vegetables from the oven and transfer to the high-powered blender and blitz to a smooth purée.

Meanwhile make the pizza base. Mix all the dry ingredients together in a large mixing bowl. Add 170 ml/3/4 cup of water and bring the dough together to form a ball and put on the prepared baking sheet.

If you have a pizza stone put it in the oven to warm up. Roll the dough into a thin 30-cm/12-inch round on the oiled baking sheet. Then once the sauce ingredients are cooked turn the oven up to 200°C (400°F) Gas 6.

Bake the base on the pizza stone by shooting it into the top of the oven from the baking sheet, or on the baking sheet, for 20 minutes, or until golden. Remove the base from the oven but keep the heat on at 180°C (350°F) Gas 4. Rub with a peeled garlic clove to infuse it with flavour.

To make the tapenade, blitz all the ingredients except the oil together in a food processor. Slowly add the oil with the motor running. Set aside.

To build the pizza, spread the pizza sauce (you made not need all of it) over the base and bake for 5–10 minutes. Mix the chicken slices with 2 tablespoons of the tapenade. Add this and the other toppings to the pizza drizzling over a little more tapenade. Bake for another 10 minutes, or until everything is piping hot, then serve.

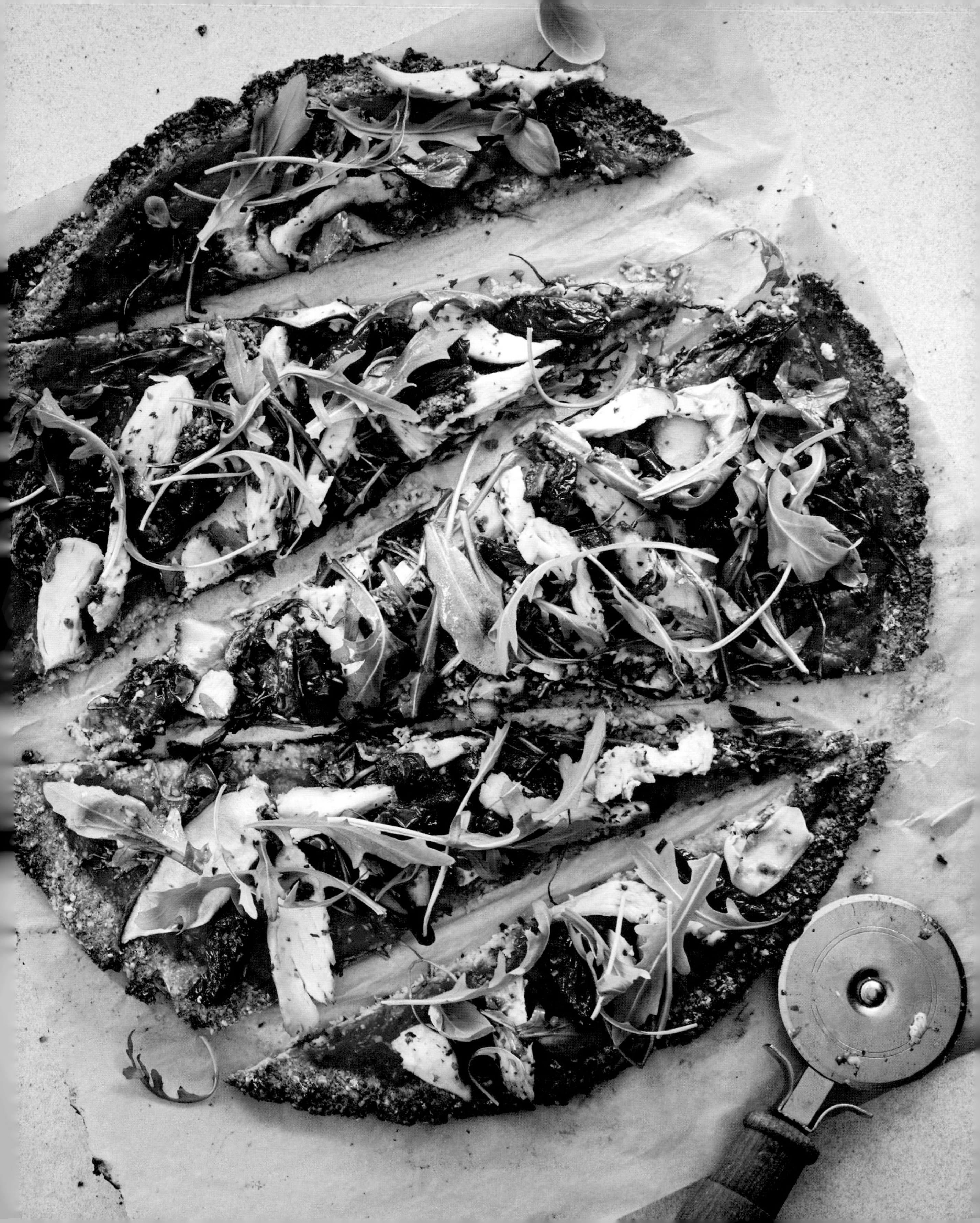

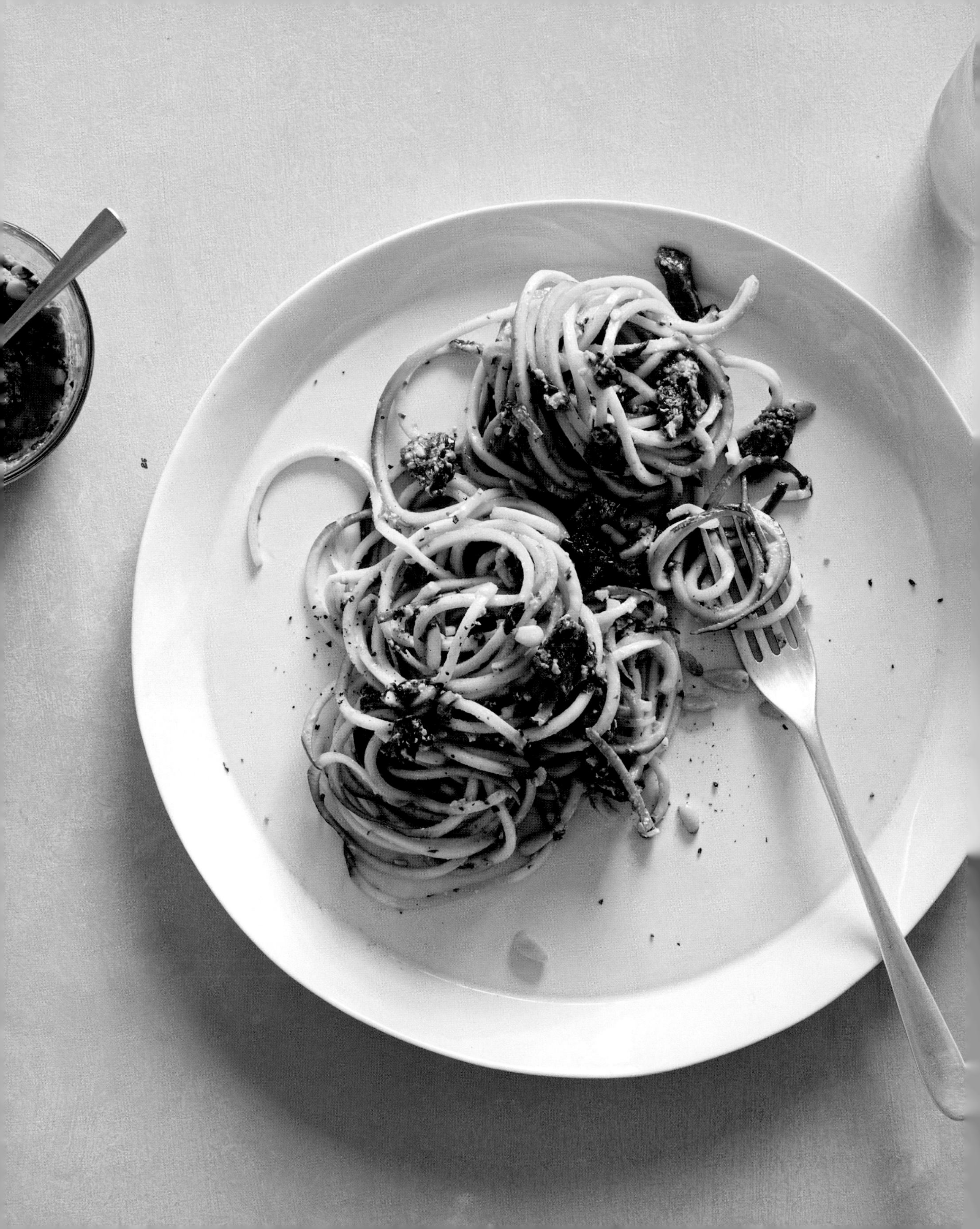

pesto 'pasta'

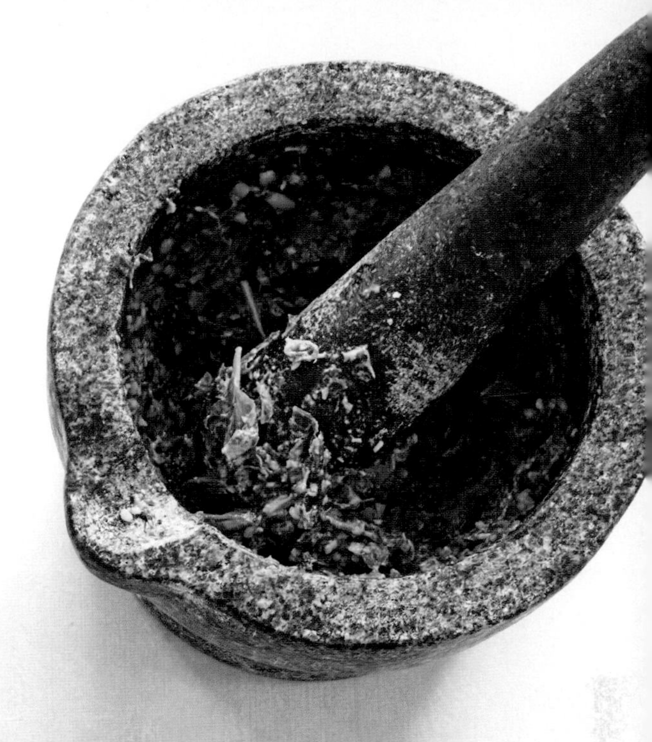

Pesto has always been one of my favourite things to add to chicken, to salads, on top of roasted vegetables, on pizzas – you name it, I've pestoed it! So a cheese-free pesto was one of the first things I made Paleo. Courgettes/zucchini are an excellent source of potassium and hold their shape well when spiralized, making them both a healthy and versatile alternative to wheat pasta.

½–1 garlic clove, to taste

2 handfuls of pine nuts

2 big handfuls of fresh basil, roughly chopped

extra virgin olive oil, to taste

a handful of sun-dried tomatoes, chopped

1 chargrilled red (bell) pepper, chopped

3–4 courgettes/zucchini

salt and black pepper, to season

SERVES 4

In a pestle and mortar crush the garlic with some whole rock salt. The salt helps break it down into a paste.

Warm the pine nuts in a dry frying pan/skillet set over low heat. I find when they are warmed they are easier to break down and release more flavour.

Add half to three-quarters of the pine nuts to the crushed garlic and set the rest aside for later. Crush to a paste. Add the basil to the pestle and mortar and grind to a paste. Add a little pepper to taste and once you are happy with the consistency of the paste, slowly add a little olive oil. The consistency of the pesto will depend on how much oil you add and this is down to personal preference.

Add the sun-dried tomatoes, chargrilled (bell) pepper and remaining nuts to the pesto and stir through.

Store in the fridge in an airtight container until ready to use. The oil acts as a preservative so depending how oil-laden you made your pesto it should keep for 2 days and up to 1 week.

Spiralize the courgettes/zucchini on the large noodle attachment. Preheat a large frying pan/skillet with 1 tablespoon of olive oil (or a little water) over medium heat and add the courgetti. Cook for 2–3 minutes until slightly softened but still al dente. Season with salt and stir through the pesto to serve.

vegetable stir-fry

Stir-fry is my go-to comfort food. I've never really been one for noodles and rice with these sorts of dishes so cutting those out to go Paleo was no problem. The texture and flavour of this dish is great and I love to use different coloured vegetables (reds, oranges, greens, yellows, purples) to make it look really appetizing.

1 red and 1 green (bell) pepper, sliced into strips

3 carrots, cut into ribbons

150 g/5 oz. green beans, sliced

100 g/5 oz. baby corn, roughly chopped (optional, omit if following strict Paleo diet, see Note)

2 pak choi/bok choy, sliced lengthways

coconut oil, for frying (optional)

black sesame seeds, to garnish

sesame oil, to drizzle

stir-fry sauce

½–1 teaspoon freshly grated ginger, to taste

½–1 green chilli/chile, thinly sliced, to taste

½ red chilli/chile, thinly sliced

1 garlic clove, finely chopped

a small handful of jarred pea aubergines/eggplants, roughly chopped

2 tablespoons pomegranate molasses

2 tablespoons liquid coconut aminos

freshly squeezed juice of 1 lime

SERVES 4

First prepare the stir-fry sauce. Mix all the ingredients together in a small bowl and set aside until ready to cook.

The hard work in this dish is in the slicing of the vegetables. Prepare the ingredients as indicated, ensuring everything is sliced or chopped in a similar way to allow the ingredients to cook at the same time.

Set a large wok or frying pan/skillet over high heat and add a little coconut oil or water. Add the vegetables and cook for 1–2 minutes until you have the desired crunch – I like my vegetables to be al dente but you can cook them for a little longer if you prefer.

Tip half of the stir-fry sauce into the pan and toss to coat. Continue to cook for 1–2 minutes longer to release the flavours of the sauce into the dish, then remove the pan from the heat.

Top the dish with black sesame seeds and drizzle with a little sesame oil. Serve immediately with the remaining stir-fry sauce on the side to pour over to taste.

Note: Baby corn is technically a cereal grain and could be left out but I like the crunch it adds to this dish. If you feel like you need an extra bit of protein, try adding king prawns/jumbo shrimp, sliced chicken or nuts.

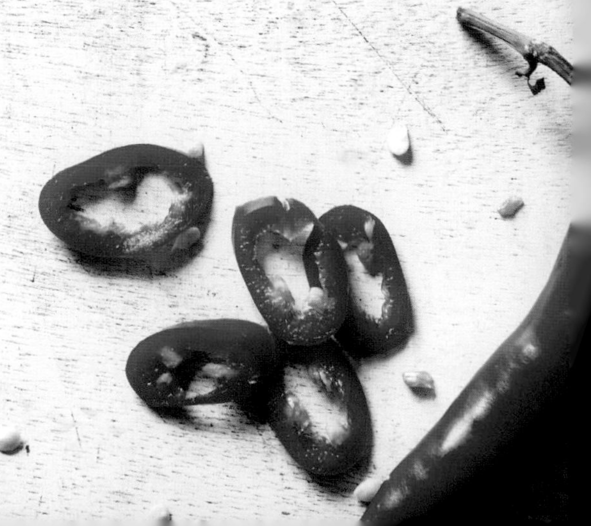

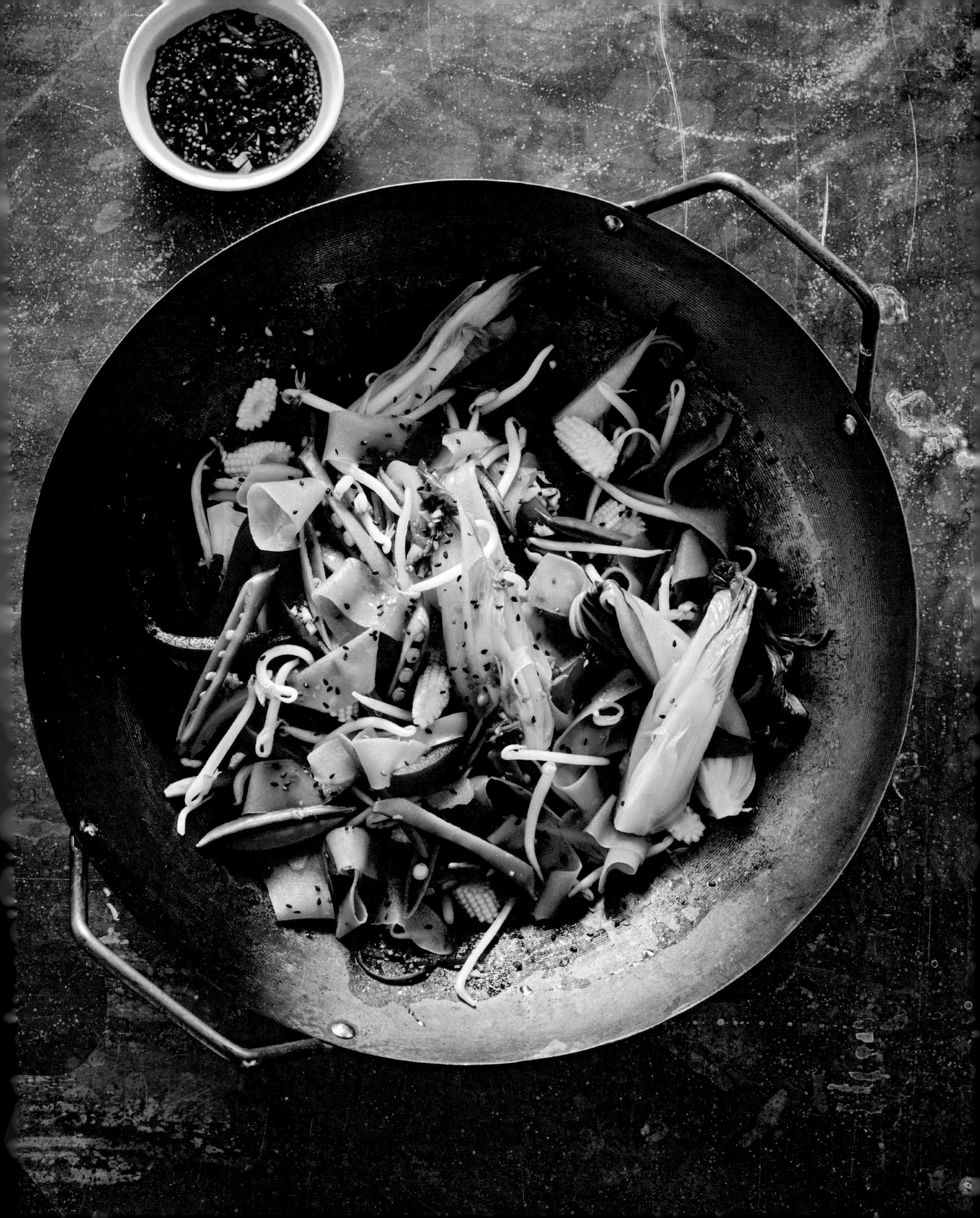

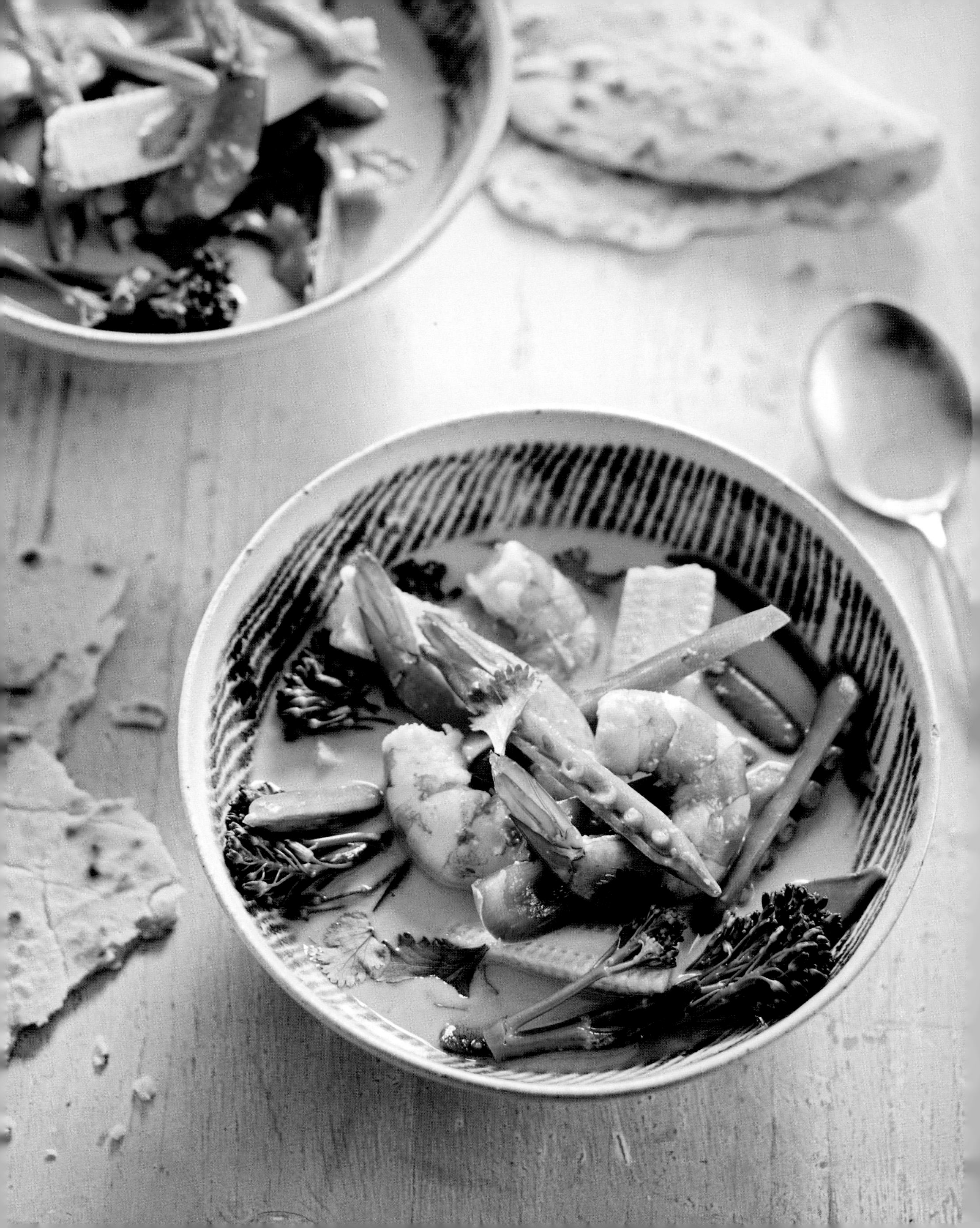

yellow seafood curry with paleo chapattis

coconut oil, for frying

250 g/9 oz. king prawns/ jumbo shrimp (heads and shells on)

1 fresh red chilli/chile, slit

4 heaped tablespoons grated creamed coconut

a 400-ml/14-oz. can coconut milk

1/2 cup mangetout/snow peas

1/2 cup sugar snap peas

1 (bell) pepper, sliced

100 g/1 cup baby corn (optional – omit if following strict Paleo diet)

100 g/4–5 stalks tenderstem broccoli

fresh coriander/cilantro leaves, to garnish

yellow curry paste

1 galangal root

a 2.5-cm/1-inch piece of fresh turmeric and a 2.5-cm/1-inch piece of fresh ginger

1/2 red onion

3 garlic cloves

1 large bay leaf

4 cardamom pods

1 teaspoon fennel seeds

1 slice cassia bark (or 1 cinnamon stick)

chapattis

160 g/scant 2 cups almond flour

240 g/2 cups arrowroot

a pinch of salt

2 tablespoons olive oil

SERVES 4

This curry paste can be used as the base for lots of different curries – I love using chicken instead of seafood, but I also love using mixed vegetables for a vegan dish. Like lots of my main meals, I advise making this the day before eating to let all the flavours infuse and strengthen in taste.

Start by blitzing the yellow curry paste ingredients together in a food processor.

Set a frying pan/skillet over medium heat and add a little coconut oil or coconut butter. Add the spice paste. Peel the shells and heads off the prawns/shrimp and add these to the spices. Keep the bodies in the fridge until ready to use. Cook for a couple minutes, then add the chilli/chile. The shells should turn pink and the flavours and smells should lift out. Fry for a further 5–10 minutes, then add the creamed coconut, coconut milk and 500 ml/2 cups of water. Cover with a lid and simmer for 20 minutes. Cool and store in fridge for at least 12 hours or overnight.

The next day, to make the chapattis, mix together the almond flour, arrowroot and salt in a large mixing bowl. Make a well in the centre then add the oil and 140 ml/scant 2/3 cup of water. Mix well and bring together into a ball. The dough should be easy to handle without being too sticky.

Pull the dough into four equal parts and roll each part into a ball. Using an oiled rolling pin, roll each ball out relatively thin onto a lightly floured piece of baking parchment – you may need a little extra arrowroot to stop it from sticking.

Set a non-stick frying pan/skillet over medium heat and brush with a little oil. The pan needs to be almost dry, so don't get carried away with the oil.

Using the baking parchment to lift the chapattis to the pan, cook on each side and keep warm until ready to serve, or cool and freeze immediately if not serving right away. (The chapattis can be defrosted and warmed in a dry pan.)

Gently warm the curry sauce in a large saucepan over low–medium heat – you may wish to then pass it through a fine-mesh sieve/strainer to get rid of any gritty bits. Turn the heat up then add the prawns/shrimp, cook for a few minutes until they just start to turn pink then add the remaining ingredients for the last few minutes. Keep the vegetables al dente so they stay vibrant in colour and have a little crunch.

To serve, top with fresh coriander/cilantro leaves and pile up the chapattis on the side.

'fish and chips'

4 fillets sea bream

1–2 tablespoons coconut butter, for frying

salt and black pepper, to season

lemon wedges and mayonnaise, to serve

mushy peas

300 g/2 cups fresh or frozen peas

4 tablespoons Vegetable Stock (optional, page 17)

zest and freshly squeezed juice of 1/4–1/2 lemon, to taste

a big handful each of fresh mint and parsley, chopped

a handful of capers, squeezed out and chopped

pea shoots, to garnish

celeriac chips

2 tablespoons coconut butter

a pinch of saffron (optional)

dried chilli/hot red pepper flakes, to taste (optional)

1 celeriac, peeled and cut into chips/fries

batter

75–100 g/2/3 cup arrowroot, plus a little extra for dusting

25 g/1/4 cup almond flour

1/2 teaspoon baking powder

150 ml/2/3 cup zesty and aromatic kombucha (or tonic water)

SERVES 4

A perfect alternative to the usual fish and chips. Use fresh and local fish to get the most flavour. You can make sweet potato chips, but I really like the flavour of celeriac with the sea bream. The mushy peas can be prepared in advance as they are actually a cold accompaniment to the dish.

Begin by making the mushy peas. Simmer the peas in the stock (or water will do). Once cooked (they should be vibrant in colour and still al dente), strain, and mash. Mix in the rest of the ingredients and transfer to a serving dish. Garnish with pea shoots and set aside or in the fridge until ready to serve.

Preheat the oven to 200°C (400°F) Gas 6.

For the celariac chips, warm the coconut butter in a saucepan over low heat and add the saffron (if using), salt, pepper and chilli/hot red pepper flakes if you like a little warmth. Put the celeriac chips in a baking dish and coat with the seasoned butter.

Bake in the preheated oven for roughly 15 minutes or until cooked through but golden and slightly crispy on the outside.

To prepare the battered fish, mix together the arrowroot (you may need more or less to thicken the batter once you add the liquid), almond flour, a pinch of salt and baking powder in a large mixing bowl. Stir with a fork while slowly pouring in the kombucha. (Make sure you use a fresh bottle so that it has the most fizz.) The batter should be thick but runny, smooth with no lumps. If there are lumps, you just added the kombucha too fast, pass through a fine-mesh sieve/strainer if this is the case, squash the lumps to a paste and mix with a little extra kombucha to loosen it before adding back to the batter.

Set a non-stick frying pan/skillet over medium–high heat and add the coconut butter. Lightly coat the sea bream fillets in arrowroot, dip in the batter, and carefully lay skin-side down in the hot pan, taking care so that you don't get burnt by the oil if it spatters. If the batter looks like it it cooking too fast turn down the heat a little. However you need the pan hot enough to crisp up the batter, just not burning it. It should take only a couple of minutes on each side.

Serve the fish with the celeriac chips, lemon wedges to squeeze over and mushy peas and mayonnaise on the side.

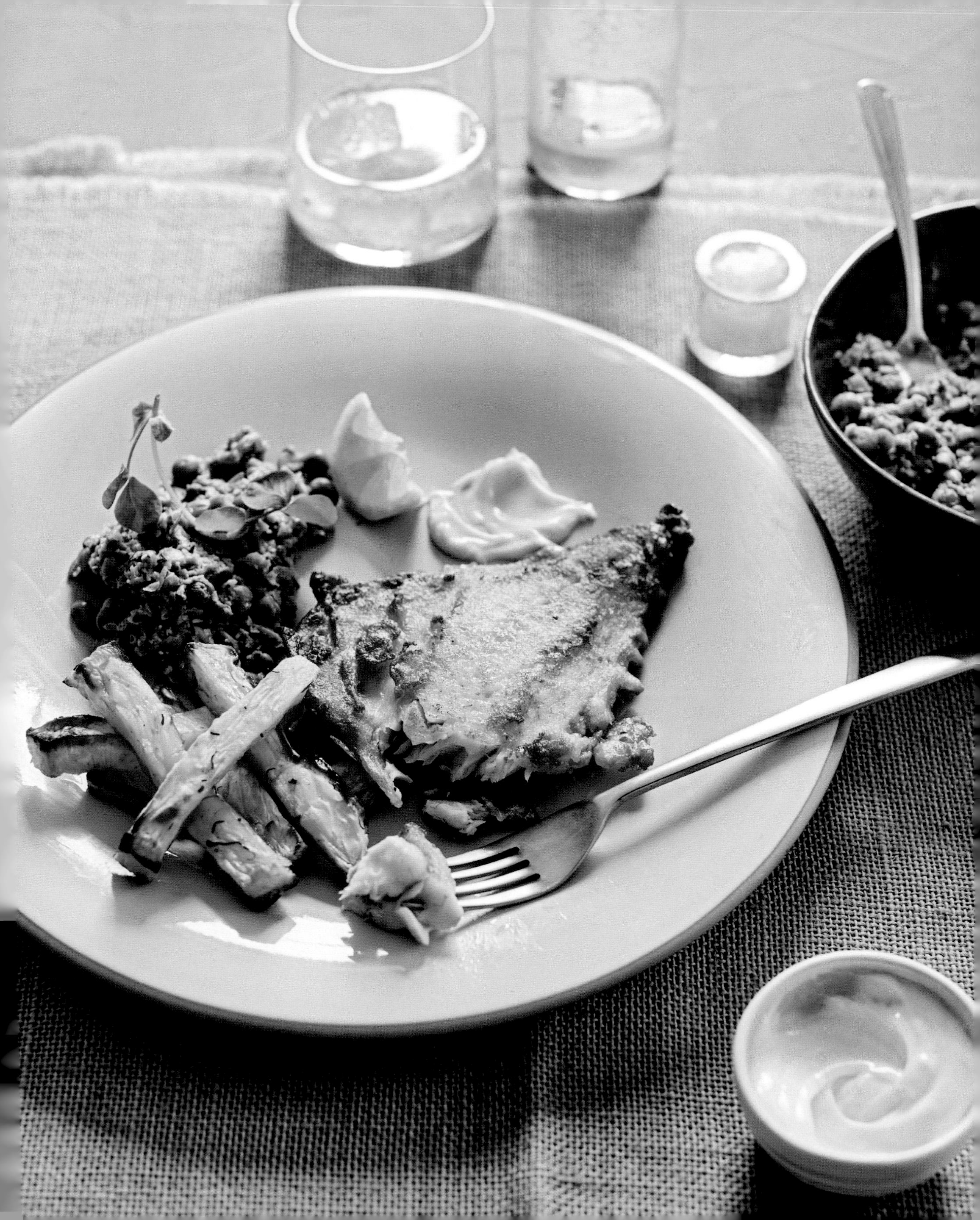

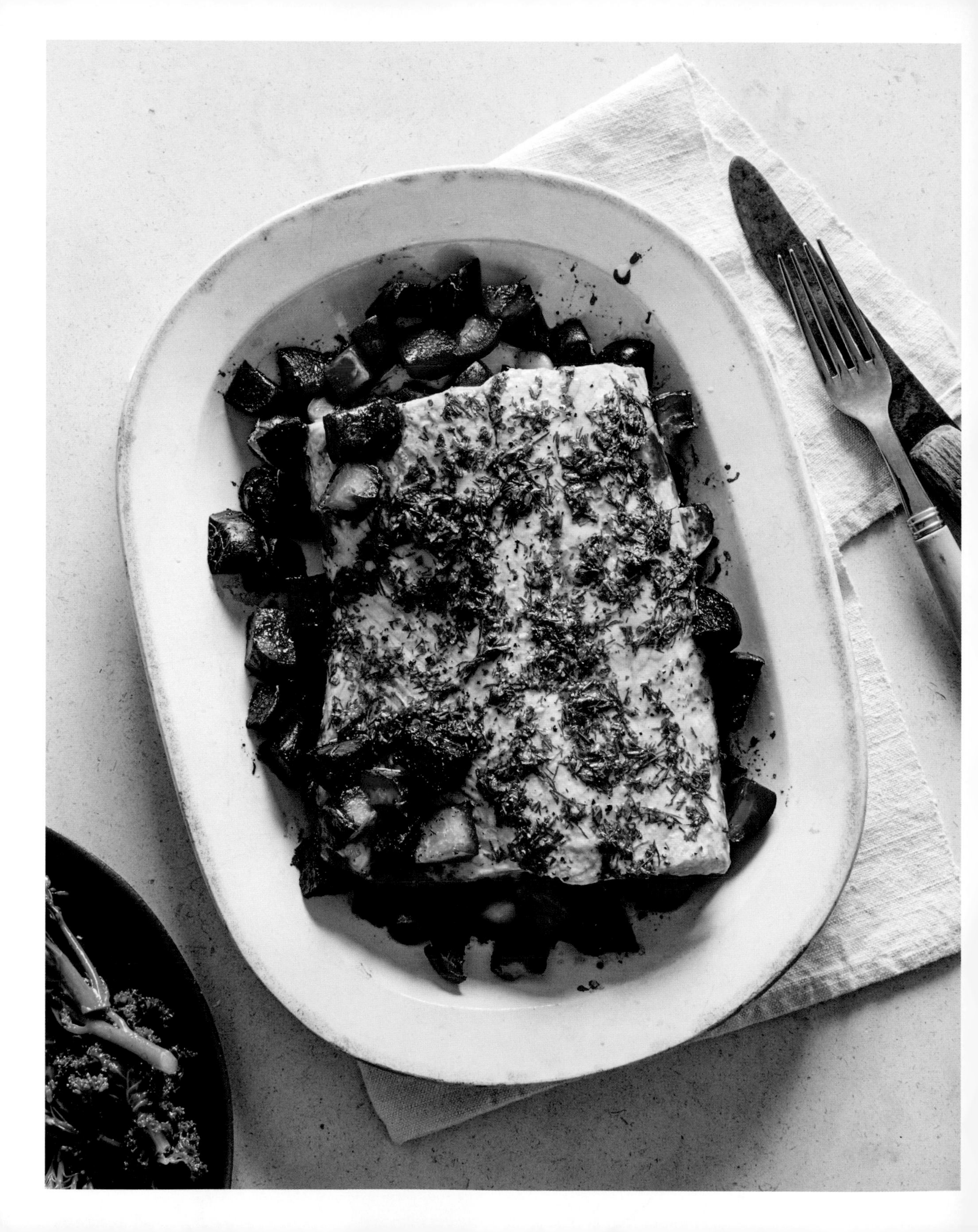

roast salmon and beetroot/beets

This dish is packed full of zingy deliciousness and nutrient-rich root veggies. I like to keep the skin on the beetroot/beets and other root vegetables because it adds an extra dimension of flavour, plus there's added goodness in those skins.

5–6 medium purple, golden or candied beetroot/beets, scrubbed clean and diced

1–3 garlic cloves, crushed

zest of 1 lemon and freshly squeezed juice of 2

2 bunches of fresh dill, roughly chopped

olive oil, to drizzle

a bunch of fresh parsley, roughly chopped

a 2.5-cm/1-inch piece of fresh ginger, grated

1 side of salmon

salt and black pepper, to season

to serve (optional)

blanched and sautéed tenderstem broccoli, dark leafy greens and samphire

SERVES 4

Preheat the oven to 180°C (350°F) Gas 4.

Mix the beetroot/beets together with the garlic, lemon zest and 1 bunch of dill in a baking dish. Drizzle with olive oil and season with salt and pepper. Bake in the preheated oven for 20 minutes.

Meanwhile, mix together the lemon juice, chopped parsley, second bunch of dill, a pinch of pepper, ginger and a little olive oil.

Remove the dish from the oven and push the beetroot/beet cubes to the sides to make room for the salmon. Lay the salmon skin-side down in the dish, pour over the lemon and herb dressing, saving a little to dress the plate to serve.

Return to the oven and bake for another 15 minutes, or until the salmon is cooked through, then serve.

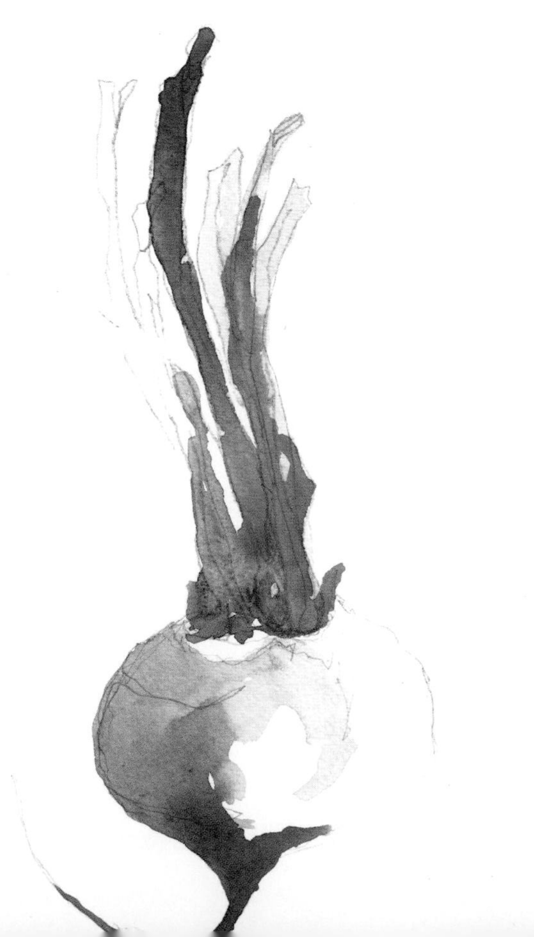

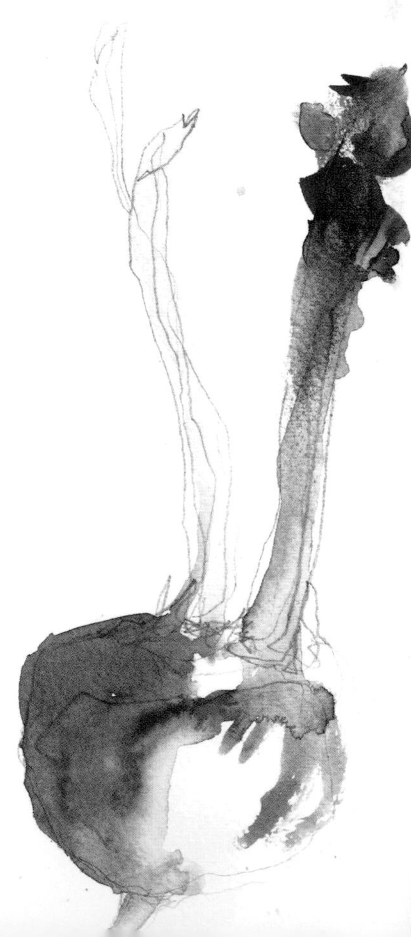

beef and oxtail ragù with spiralized sweet potato

I try to use different cuts of meat in cooking including the oxtail here. Toby from Pure Taste used to cook with all sorts of interesting cuts – I really admire the way he works. His pig's head terrine is something I never thought I would enjoy, but it's divine!

beef dripping, for cooking
600 g/21 oz. oxtail (on the bone)
600 g/21 oz. beef short rib
arrowroot, to coat
3 smoked garlic cloves, finely chopped
2 carrots, finely diced
1 large white onion, finely diced
2 celery stalks/ribs, finely diced
2 fresh rosemary sprigs
2 bay leaves
400 ml/1¾ cups chicken stock (or water)
1½ teaspoons wholegrain mustard
3 tablespoons good-quality balsamic vinegar
225 g/8 oz. baby plum tomatoes
salt and black pepper, to season

to serve
2–3 large sweet potatoes
chopped fresh parsley
mixed green salad

SERVES 4–6

Set a large casserole dish over medium heat and add 1–2 tablespoons of beef dripping. Coat the meat in arrowroot and sprinkle with salt and pepper. Add the meat to the dish – any fatty bits need to take priority on the heat. Once the meat is coloured and sealed, remove from the pan.

Put all the vegetables and herbs except the tomatoes in the dish and sauté for a few minutes. Return the meat to the pan, stir everything together, add the stock, mustard and balsamic, and cover with a lid. Simmer for 40 minutes.

Remove the lid and stir everything together. Cover the dish with baking parchment, and simmer over low–medium heat for another 1–2 hours, stirring occasionally. If the ragù sauce is reducing too much, add a little water and put the lid over the baking parchment.

Add the tomatoes for the last 30–40 minutes.

The meat should fall apart and fall off the bone; the sauce should be reduced and thickened. Remove the bones from the dish and keep warm.

Spiralize the sweet potato. Set a frying pan/skillet over medium heat and sauté the sweet potato with a little water for a few minutes until softened.

Serve the sweet potato with the ragù, sprinkled with chopped fresh parsley, and a side salad.

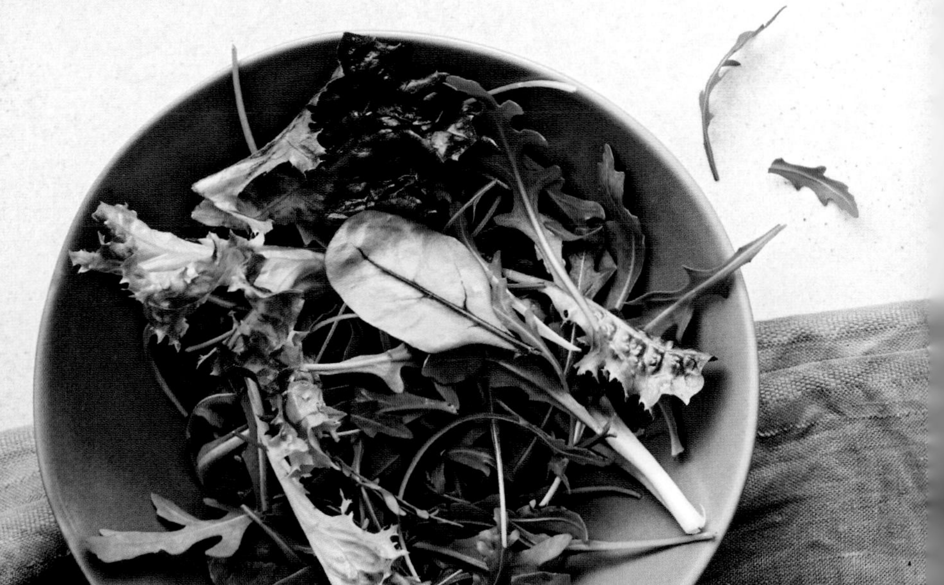

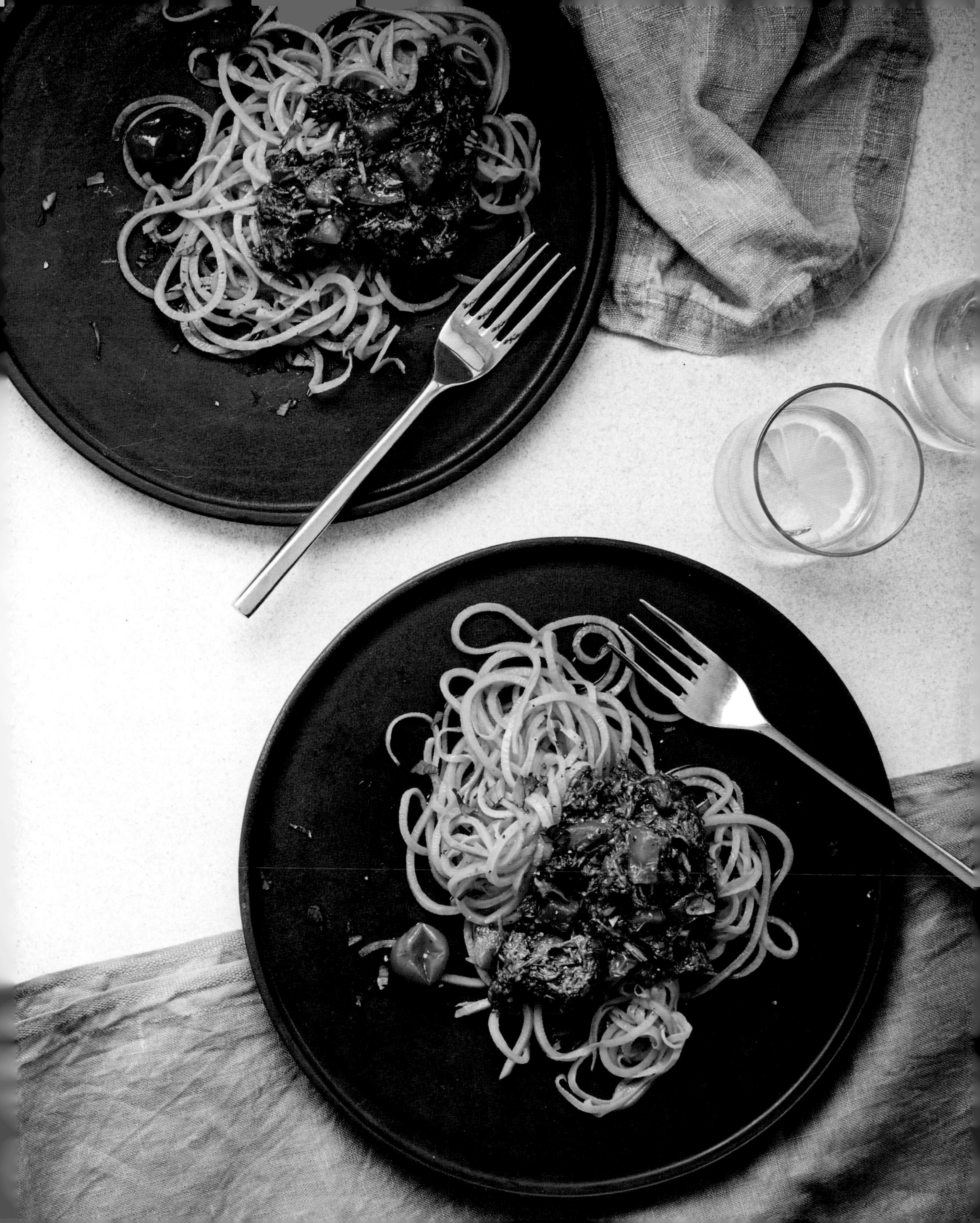

alternative roast beef dinner

I really enjoy this dinner as it's lighter than your normal Sunday roast. I love to use the leftover beef with the remoulade on an open sandwich (page 73). The Yorkshire pudding batter also makes great crêpes!

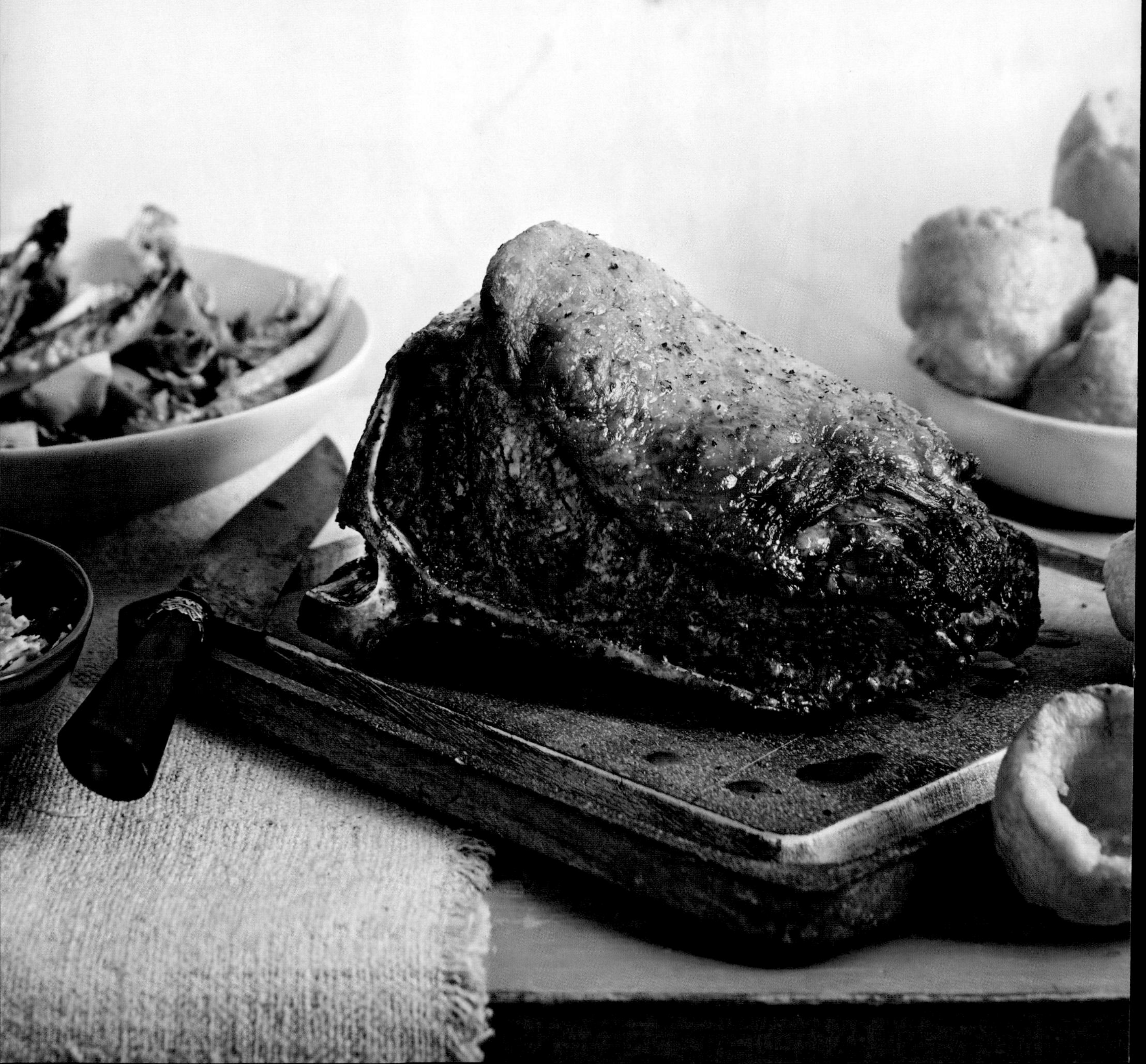

1.6 kg/3 1/2 lbs. beef joint (rib wing)

2 Little Gem/Bibb lettuces, quartered

olive oil, to drizzle

salt and black pepper, to season

Yorkshire puddings

100 g/3/4 cup arrowroot

a pinch of salt

2 eggs

100 ml/1/3 cup almond milk

beef dripping (or goose fat), for cooking

parsnip remoulade

300 g/10 1/2 oz. parsnips, grated

freshly squeezed juice of 1/2 lemon

freshly grated horseradish, to taste

a handful of fresh parsley, roughly chopped

1 1/2 teaspoons wholegrain mustard

3 tablespoons mayonnaise

1 small beetroot/beet, cut into thin strips

a 12-hole muffin pan

SERVES 4-6

Preheat the oven to 220°C (425°F) Gas 7.

Dry the skin of the beef joint with paper towels and season with a little salt and pepper, and put the joint in a roasting pan (fat-side up) in the preheated oven for 25 minutes. Baste with the fat in the pan then turn the heat down to 200°C (400°F) Gas 6 and cook for a further 10 minutes for rare beef, or longer if desired. Remove from the oven, cover loosely with foil and rest for 20 minutes. I like to keep any excess fat for other cooking purposes. After your meal you can also keep the beef bone to make a bone broth (page 17).

To make the Yorkshire puddings, mix together arrowroot and salt in a large mixing bowl. In a separate bowl, beat the eggs and almond milk. Pour into the bowl with the arrowroot, a little at a time, and whisk constantly. You want the mixture to be smooth with no lumps. Transfer to a jug/pitcher and set aside while you heat the beef dripping or oil. I find you can make this mix a few hours before and store in the fridge. Preheat the oven between 200°C (400°F) Gas 6 and 220°C (425°F) Gas 7 – precisely which temperature depends how vicious your oven is. Spoon about 1/4–1/2 teaspoon of solid beef dripping into each pan hole. It needs to be roughly 5-mm/1/4-inch deep once it's been in the oven and melted. If there isn't enough oil in the pan your Yorkshire puddings won't dip in the middle, too much oil and they won't crisp properly. It takes a little practise to get them spot on so don't worry if they aren't perfect first time – they will still taste delicious. Put the pan in the oven for about 5 minutes. The dripping or oil needs to be hot but not sizzling. Carefully pour in the batter so that it comes roughly one-third up the depth of the pan holes – the oil should still cover the top of the batter. Return the pan to the oven for 15–20 minutes, or until the Yorkshire puddings are golden brown and well risen.

To make the parsnip remoulade, put the grated parsnip in a large mixing bowl, squeeze over the lemon juice and grate over a little horseradish – you can add as much or as little as you like. Mix all the ingredients except the beetroot/beet together, then scatter the beetroot/beet through the mixture so that the white and pink colours don't completely merge together. Set aside.

To braise the lettuce, preheat a griddle pan over medium heat and put the lettuce cut-side down into the pan. Cook for a few minutes until lightly brown underneath and arrange on serving plates. Drizzle with a little olive oil.

Slice the rested beef and arrange on the plates. Serve with a Yorkshire pudding or two on each plate and the parsnip remoulade and braised lettuce on the side.

on-the-bone lamb tagine with tzatziki

I always, always, always make this dish at least one day before eating, because the flavours need time to infuse and develop. Ask the butcher for a good-quality cut of meat – I use square-cut shoulder of lamb, which I get from my butcher who is in fact my uncle. Cooked on the bone, the lamb makes its own stock while cooking. All the goodness and flavour is soaked into the meat as it cooks to make it particularly moist.

a shoulder of lamb

4–5 garlic cloves, halved

1–2 fresh rosemary sprigs

1 kg/2¼ lbs. fresh ripe tomatoes, quartered

a 2.5-cm/1-inch piece of fresh ginger

1 cinnamon stick

2 teaspoons ground turmeric

2 teaspoons cumin seeds

1 teaspoon fennel seeds

1 teaspoon medium curry powder

a small pinch of dried chilli/hot red pepper flakes

coarse sea salt and black pepper, to season

to serve

chopped fresh parsley

mixed green salad

Chapattis (page 91)

Tzatziki (page 15)

slow cooker (optional)

SERVES 4–6

To prepare the lamb, cut incisions into the fat and insert cut cloves of garlic and rosemary sprigs into the incisions. Season well with coarse sea salt and black pepper. Set a large casserole dish over medium heat and seal the meat until slightly brown. Remove the lamb and set aside.

Put all of the remaining ingredients into the dish and simmer for 20–30 minutes, stirring occasionally. Add 500 ml/2 cups of water about halfway through the cooking process.

Add the lamb and spoon the sauce over. Simmer for a further 30 minutes, then transfer everything to a slow cooker and cook for at least 9 hours. Turn the lamb every hour or so to that the sauce gets over all the meat. The sauce will thicken and slightly reduce as the lamb and the bone marinate and cook in it. If you are concerned that the sauce is reducing too much then add an extra 250 ml/1 cup of water. Once cooked, remove the bone, pull a fork through the meat to break it down so that the meat and the sauce become one and it's ready to serve. This is the best way to cook melt-in-the-mouth meat! Alternatively, cook in a casserole dish in the oven at 150°C (300°F) Gas 2 for 3–4 hours.

Serve the tagine sprinkled with chopped fresh parsley and accompanied by a mixed salad, chapattis and the tzatziki.

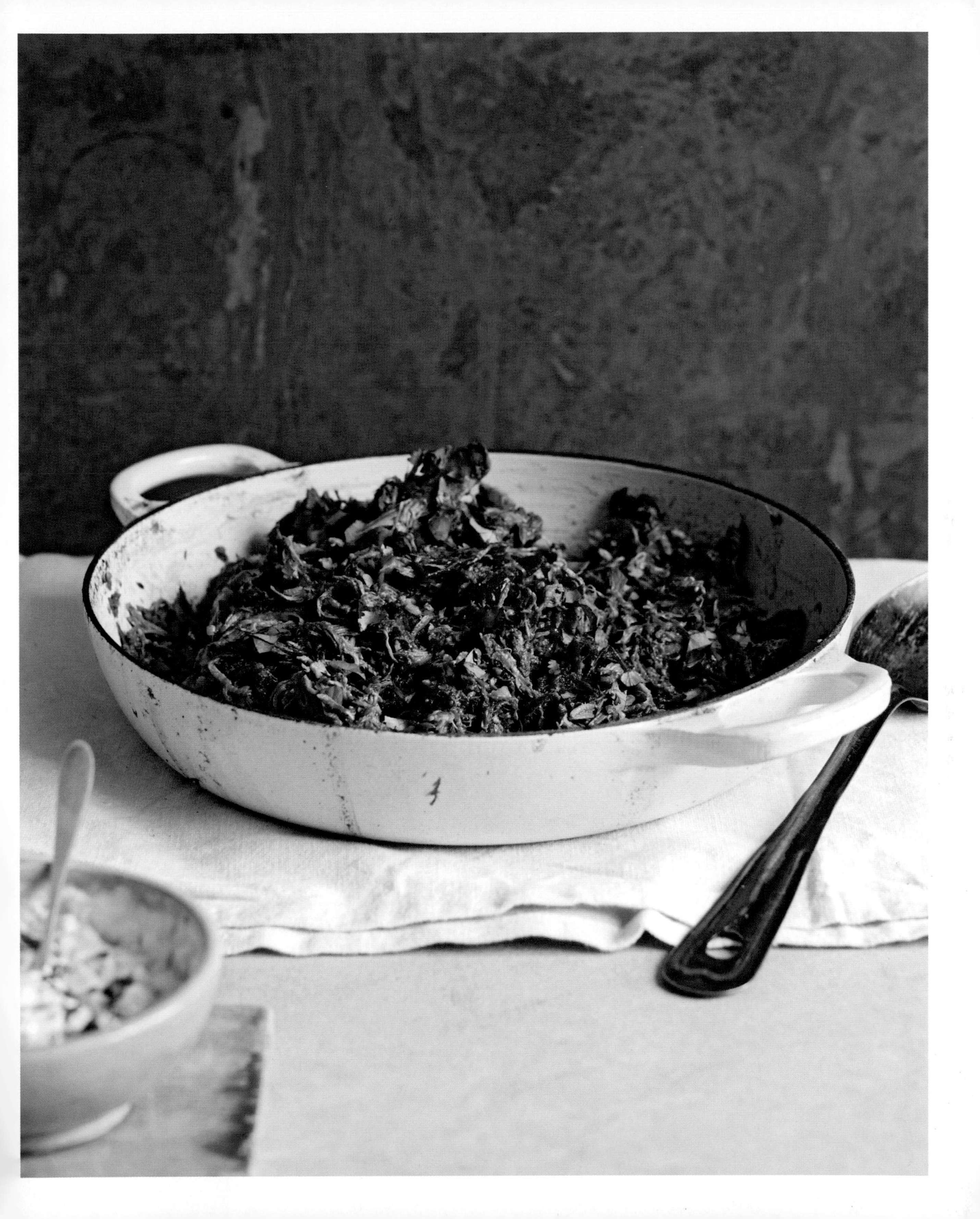

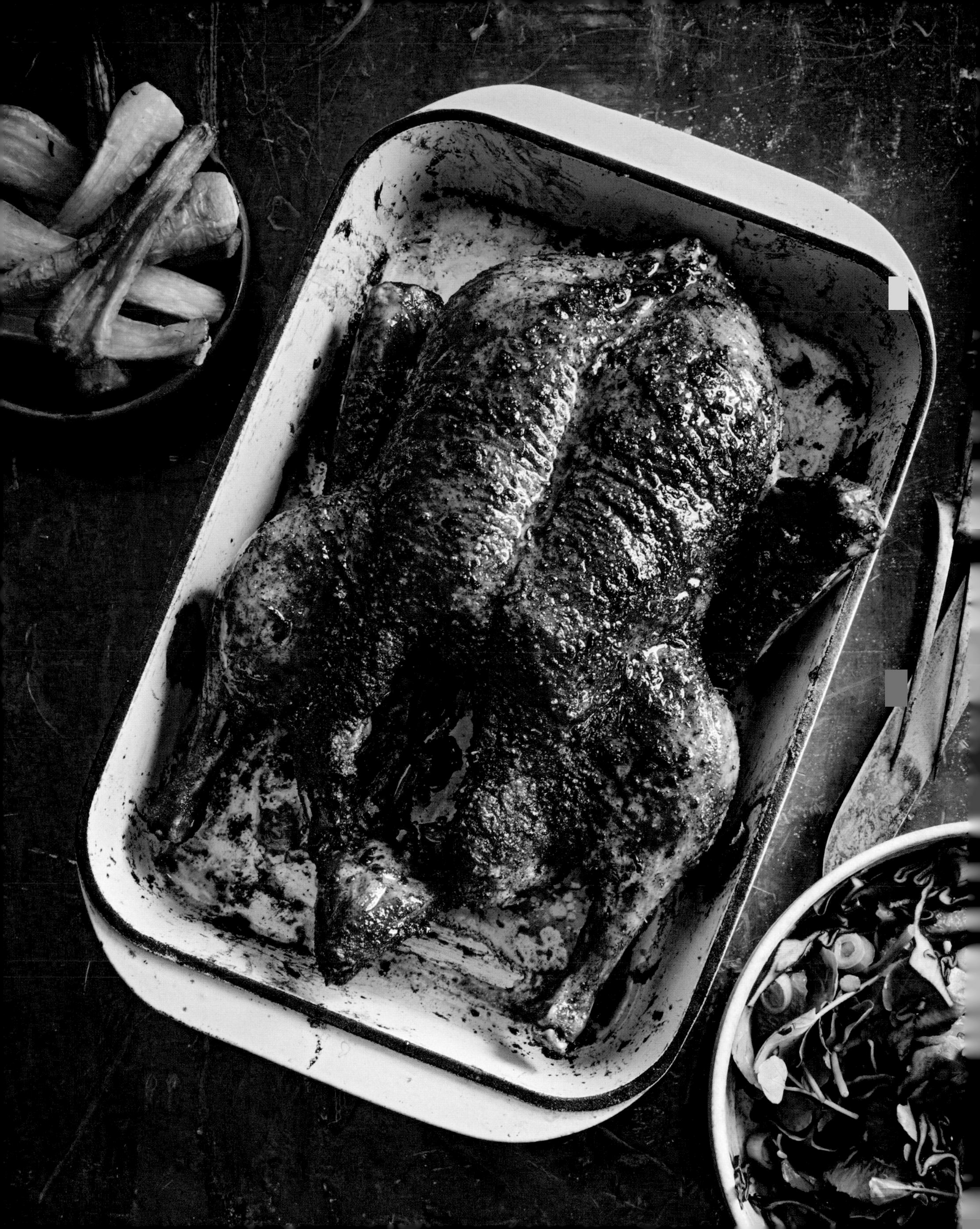

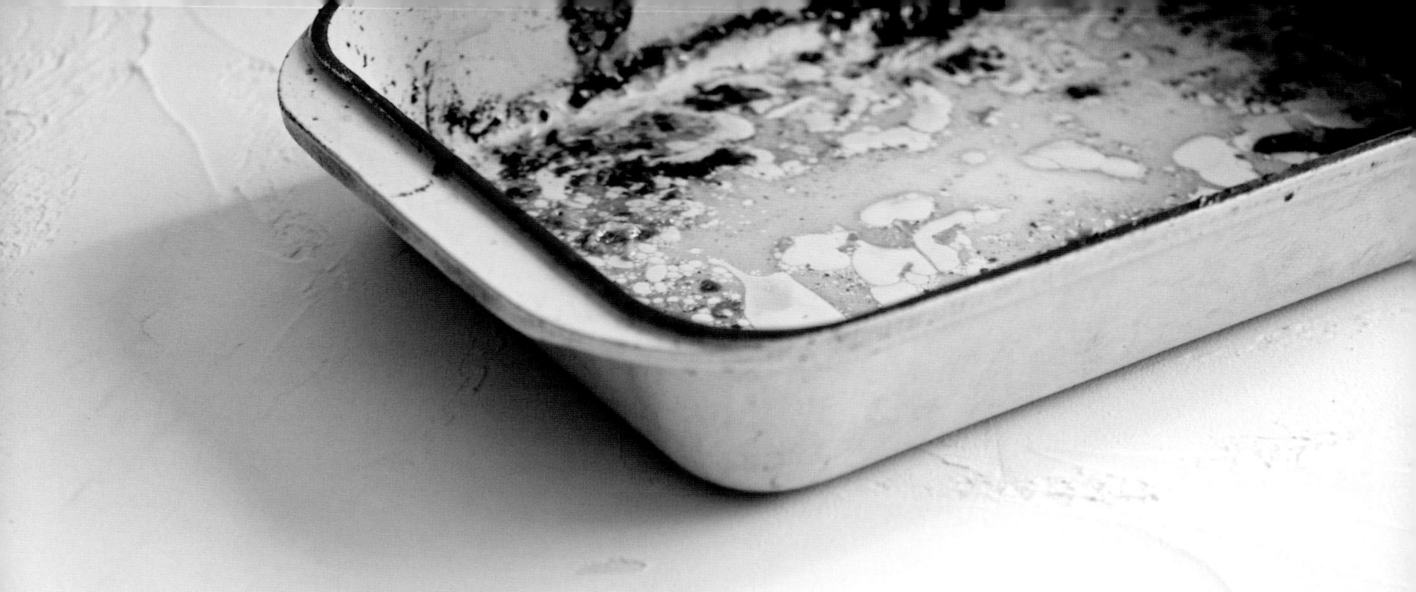

roast duck with cabbage salad

This Asian-spiced roast duck is a real indulgence. The rich duck meat can be shredded at the table to serve with the citrus-soaked cabbage for a satisfying and healthy main meal. If the salad doesn't quite cut it, add some parsnips or other root vegetables to the roasting pan with the duck and serve as an extra side.

1 whole duck

1 orange, zested then thickly sliced

Chinese five-spice and coarse sea salt or sea salt flakes, to season

cabbage salad

½ red cabbage, cored and thinly shredded

2 big handfuls of watercress

4 spring onions/scallions, roughly chopped

1 orange, zested and segmented (see Note)

balsamic vinegar and extra virgin olive oil, to drizzle

SERVES 4

Preheat the oven to 200°C (400°F) Gas 6.

Put the duck in a large roasting pan and sprinkle with orange zest and generous amounts of Chinese five-spice and sea salt. Massage into the skin, then lay the orange slices underneath the duck.

Roast uncovered in the preheated oven for 20 minutes, then turn the heat down to 180°C (350°F) Gas 4 and cook for a further 40 minutes. Remove from the oven and baste with the duck fat that has been released in the pan.

Mix all the cabbage salad ingredients except the balsamic vinegar and oil together in a large bowl. Drizzle with a little balsamic and oil as desired. Season with salt and black pepper to taste and serve with the roast duck.

Note: I find the best way to segment the orange (or any round citrus fruit) is to 'top and tail' the skin, using a knife to cut away the skin. You can then run the knife between each segment to release them from the pith. Keep the leftover skin and scraps to squeeze over the dish.

smoky pork belly with mustard slaw

For this recipe, I use pork belly still on the bone, cut into portions. It's technically a giant rib, with extra meat and crackling. Absolutely the best of both worlds! The sauce it is cooked in works well smothered on roast root veg or chicken, and any leftovers taste amazing in a wrap. Slaw is a very good friend to the Paleo eater. Fresh vegetables are transformed with a lick of dressing to jazz up simple roasts.

4 pork belly cuts (on the bone)

Mustard Slaw (page 15), to serve

smoky sauce

1 red onion, roughly chopped

4 garlic cloves, thinly sliced

4 heaped tablespoons tomato purée/paste

4 tablespoons pure maple syrup

2 tablespoons white wine vinegar

1 tablespoon black strap molasses or treacle

2 tablespoons olive oil

a few dashes of liquid coconut aminos, to taste

freshly squeezed juice of 1/2 lemon

chilli powder and smoked paprika, to taste

salt and black pepper, to season

SERVES 4

Preheat the oven to 200°C (400°F) Gas 6.

To prepare the pork belly, score the skin and rub sea salt all over. Lay in a roasting pan with the skin facing up, making sure the edges don't touch the sides or you won't get proper crackling. Roast in the preheated oven for 20 minutes.

While the pork is in the oven prepare the smoky sauce. Add all the ingredients to a saucepan and set over low–medium heat. Cook for a few minutes until the onions and garlic are cooked. Then use a handheld electric blender to blend all the ingredients with enough water to bind them together.

Remove the pork from the oven and baste with the oil that has been released from it. Pour any excess oil out of the pan and reserve for use in another recipe.

Turn the heat down to 170°C (325°F) Gas 3 and return the pork to cook for a further 20 minutes.

Brush the pork with a generous amount of sauce so every 'rib belly' is covered but you still have about half of the mixture.

Cook for 25 minutes more, brushing over with more sauce towards the end.

Remove the pork from the oven and brush over a little extra sauce if needed. Keep any remaining sauce in a sterilized glass jar in the fridge.

Enjoy the ribs with the mustard slaw on the side or shred the meat off the bone and layer up in a wrap with a mound of slaw on top.

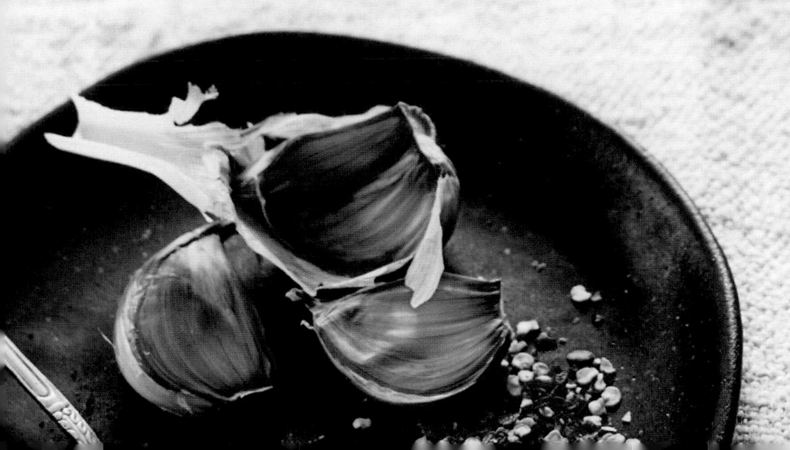

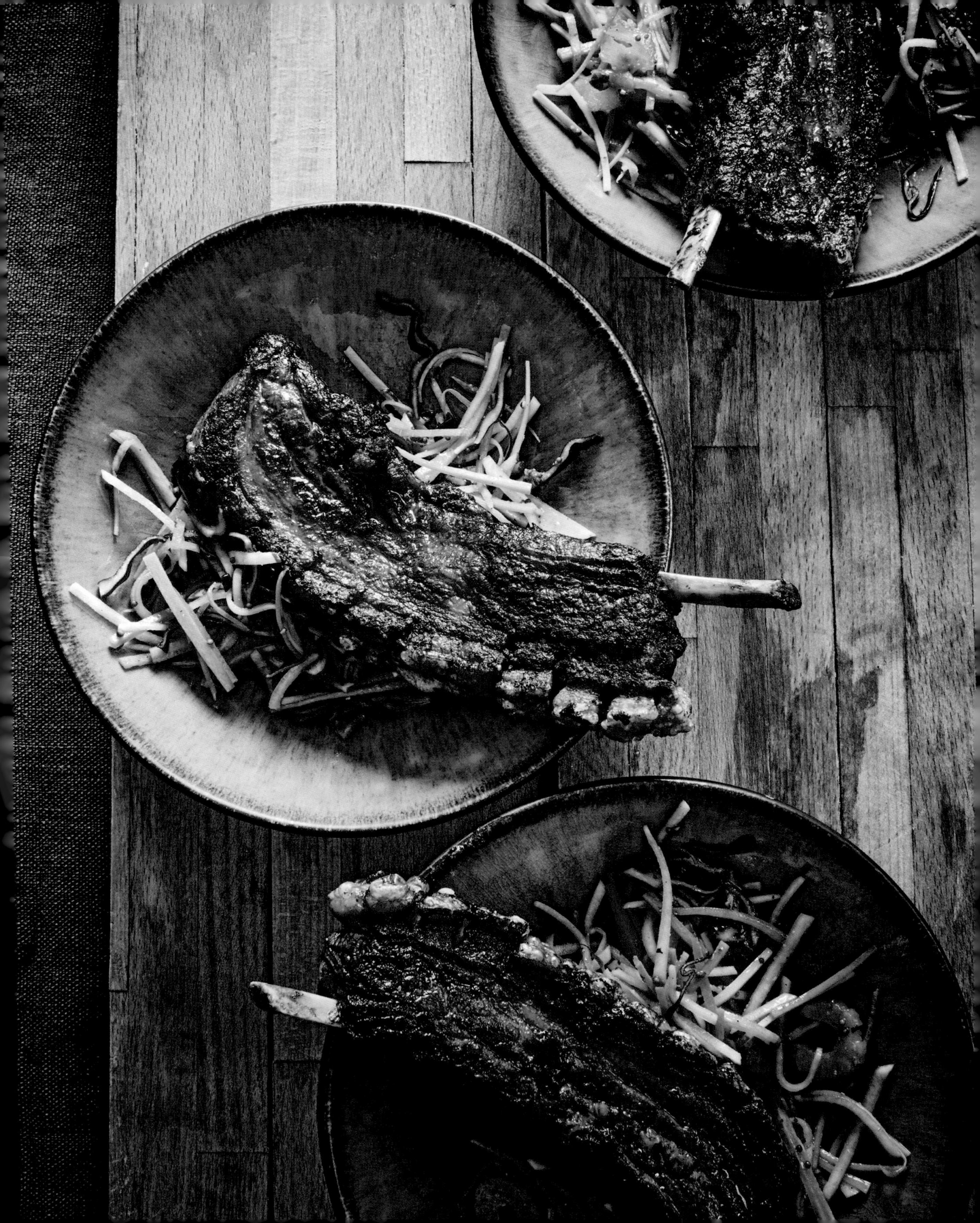

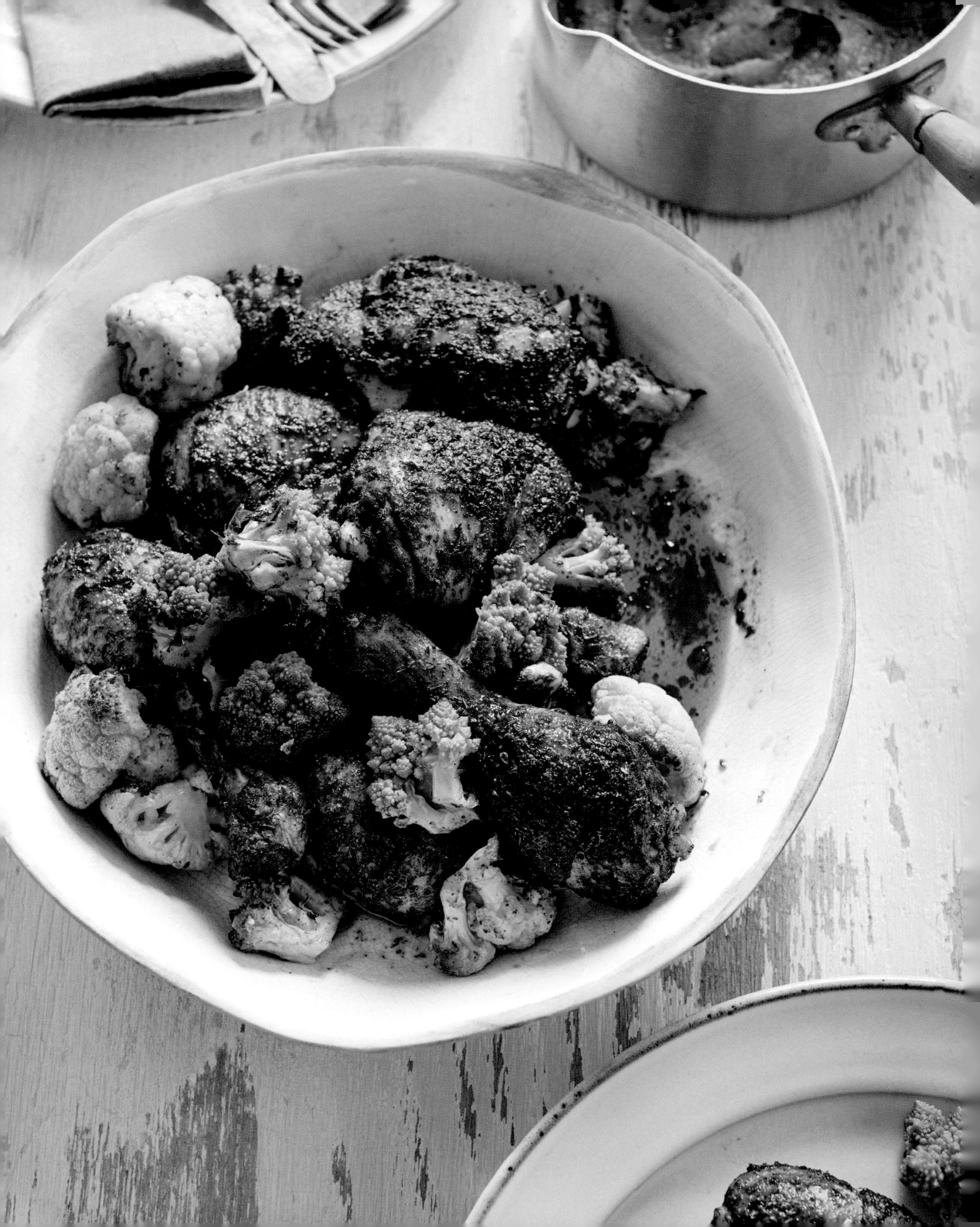

chicken pieces with carrot and squash purée

I highly recommend having a well-stocked spice cupboard. When writing this chicken recipe I took a lucky dip from my spice collection and tweaked the flavours until I was happy.

4 chicken thighs (skin on)

4 chicken drumsticks (skin on)

1 heaped tablespoon ground cumin

3/4 tablespoon mild chilli powder

1 teaspoon ground ginger

1 1/2 teaspoons paprika

1 heaped teaspoon ground cinnamon

1 tablespoon dried marjoram

salt and black pepper, to season

cooking oil of choice (I like duck fat)

1 head of broccoli (or cauliflower), cut into florets

cavolo nero, steamed to serve (optional)

carrot and squash purée

1 medium butternut squash, peeled and diced

4 carrots, diced

1 onion, diced

2 teaspoons black onion seeds

2 teaspoons ground coriander

a 400-ml/14-oz. can coconut milk

100 ml/1/3 cup Vegetable Stock (optional, page 17)

1 garlic clove

a 2-cm/3/4-inch piece of fresh turmeric, peeled and sliced

SERVES 4

First make the purée. Put all the ingredients in a saucepan and cover with a lid. Bring to a simmer over medium heat and cook for 20 minutes then remove the lid and cook until the butternut squash is soft and carrots are cooked but still slightly firmer.

Strain and leave the veg to drain for a few minutes, then transfer back to the saucepan and blend with a handheld electric blender.

Preheat the oven to 180°C (350°F) Gas 4.

Pat the chicken skin dry with paper towels and put the chicken thighs and drumsticks in a large baking dish.

Mix all the spices together and season with salt and pepper. Coat the chicken in the spice mixture and rub with the oil of your choice. Use your hands to really coat each piece of chicken in the spices.

Roast in the preheated oven for 15–20 minutes until the skin starts to crisp.

Add the broccoli florets to the baking dish and roast for another 15–20 minutes until the chicken is cooked. The broccoli should be al dente.

Serve with the carrot and squash purée and steamed cavolo nero if desired.

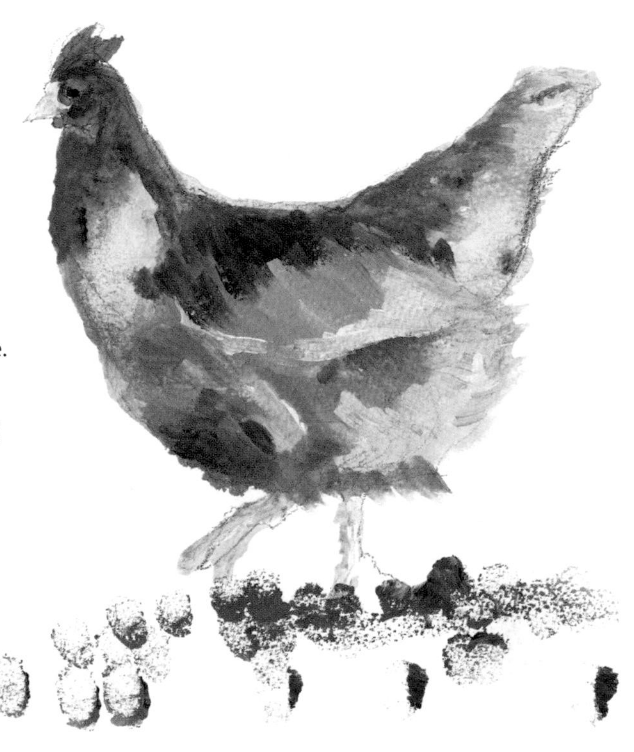

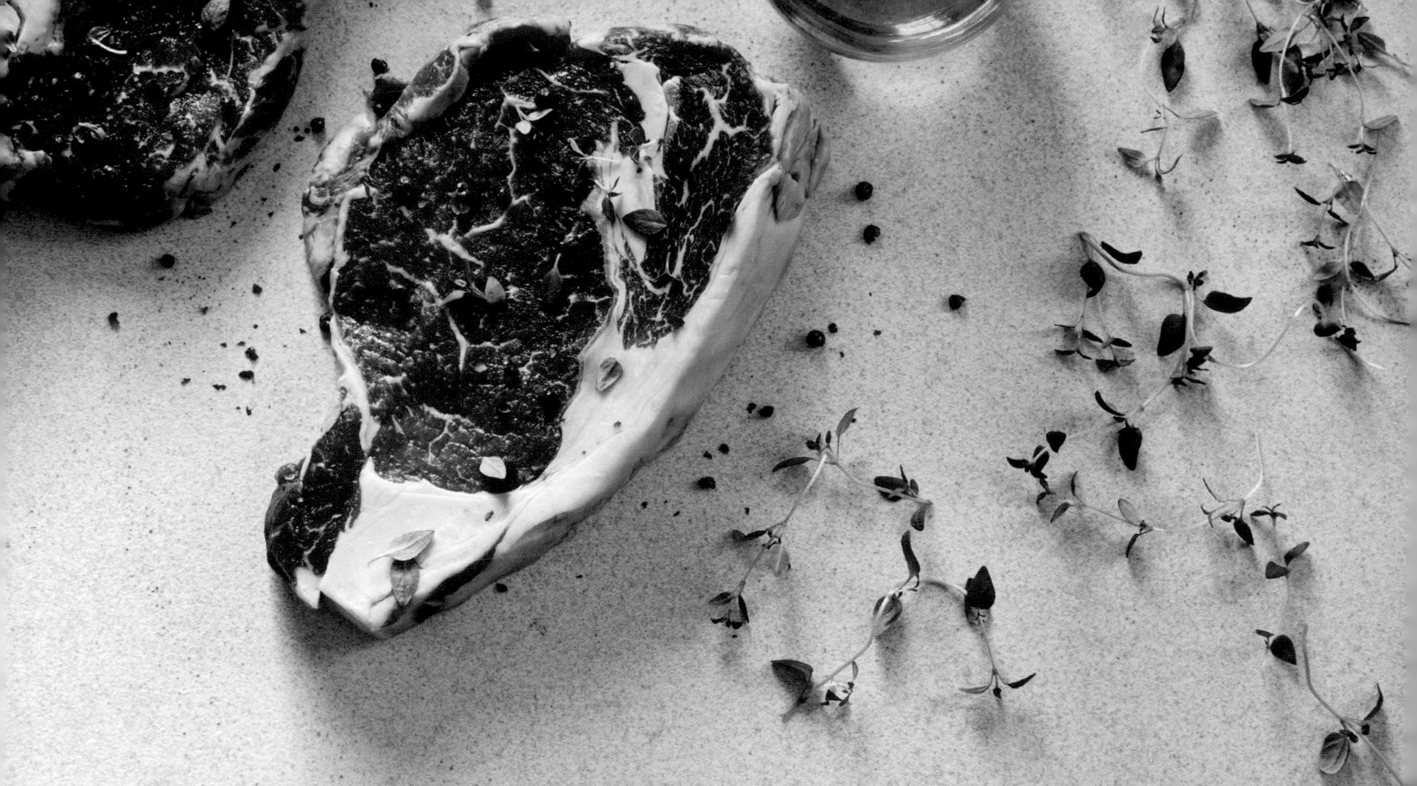

lemon thyme and pink peppercorn steak

Simple and easy, this steak supper is a great way to get a protein fix at the end of a long day. Buy the best quality meat you can afford – the better the steak the more delicious the meal.

1 sweet potato, cut into wedges

1 sirloin steak

leaves from 6–10 sprigs of fresh lemon thyme, chopped

1/2–1 tablespoon pink peppercorns, crushed

olive oil, to drizzle

salt and black pepper, to season

to serve

mixed green salad

Garlic Mayo (page 14)

a baking sheet lined with baking parchment

SERVES 1

Preheat the oven to 180°C (350°F) Gas 4.

First prepare the sweet potato wedges. Spread the wedges out on the prepared baking sheet and sprinkle with a little salt. Bake in the preheated oven for 25–30 minutes, or until crisp on the outside and cooked through.

Rub the steak with generous amounts of lemon thyme and crushed pink peppercorns. Season and drizzle with a little oil. Allow the meat to come to room temperature while marinating in this mixture.

Set a griddle pan over medium–high heat until smoking hot. Sear the fat of the steak first, then cook both sides. How well you like it cooked will determine the cooking time (this is also dependant on how thick the steak is), but I like my steak medium-rare and cook it for 2 minutes on each side.

Remove the steak from the pan, pour over any juices that were released into the pan, and rest for a few minutes before serving with the sweet potato wedges. I like to have a simple mixed salad on the side with a little garlic mayonnaise to dip the sweet potato into.

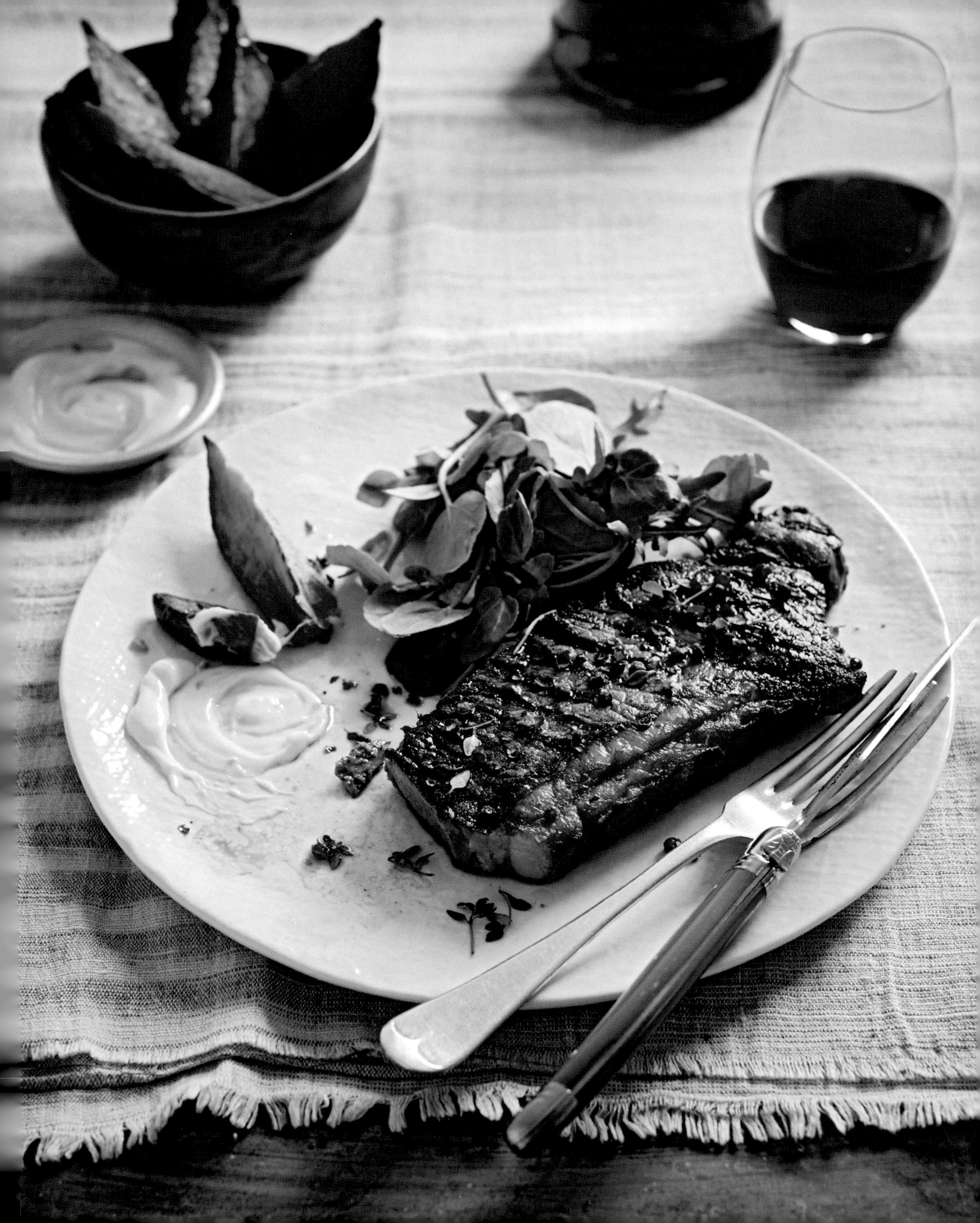

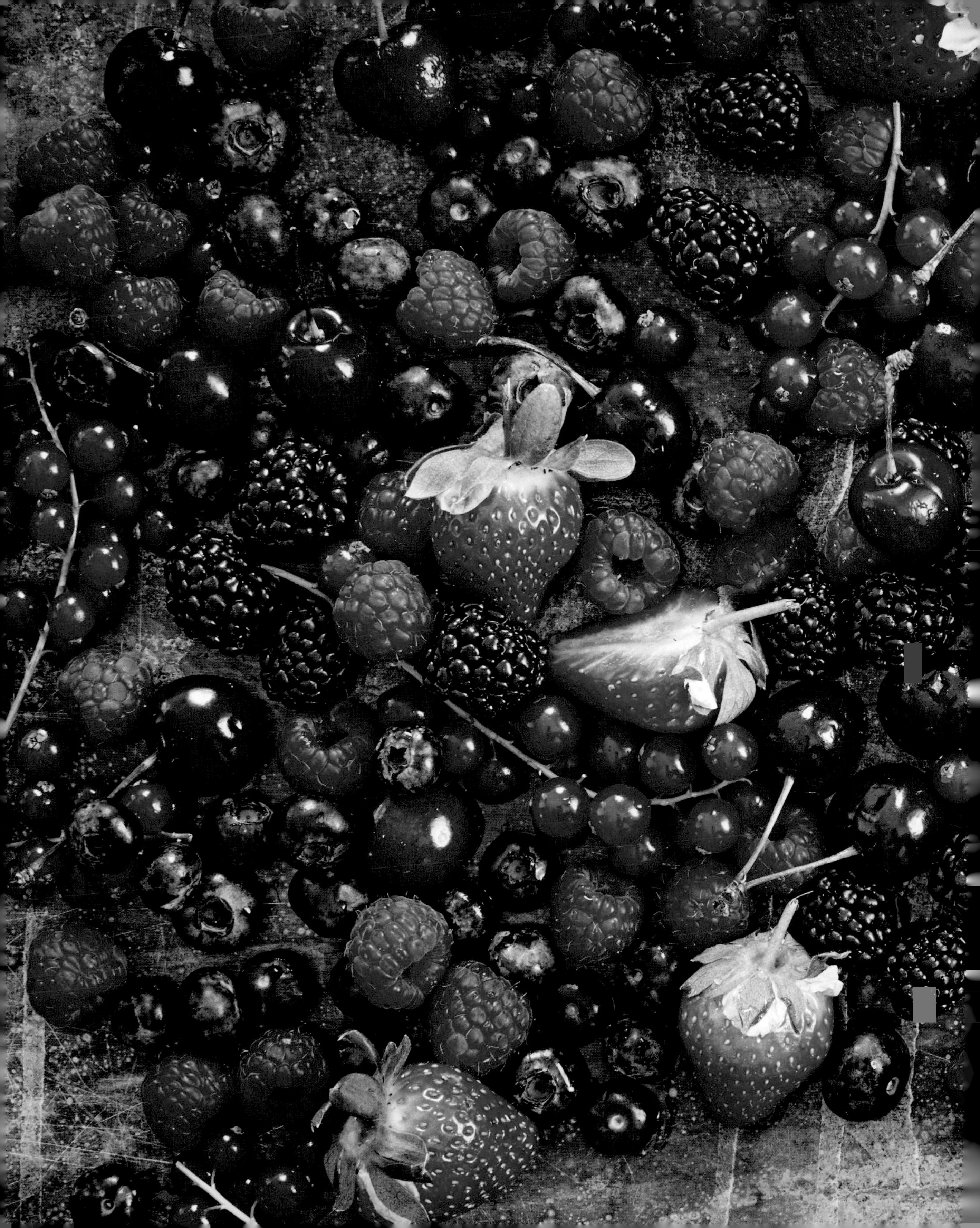

tasty treats

When you feel you need something sweet you don't have to ignore all your good eating habits. The recipes in this chapter will give you enough options to enable you to stick to the Paleo ingredients list (page 11) and still have your indulgent treat. I guarantee that you won't have to fall off the Paleo wagon!

strawberry and gooseberry trifle

I wrote this recipe while I was working at Pure Taste restaurant. The best thing about it is that you can adjust or change the fruit used to make all manner of different types of layered dessert. It uses half of the cake in the Victoria Sponge on page 131 so you could even use up leftover cake or just bake one of the layers fresh.

5 tablespoons coconut oil

75 g/1/2 cup coconut cream (the solidified coconut from a can of coconut milk or cream, see Note, page 15)

3 eggs

100 g/3 1/2 oz. palm sugar

1/2 teaspoon pure vanilla extract

2 1/2 tablespoons coconut flour

1 tablespoon tapioca flour

1 teaspoon baking powder

1–2 handfuls of blackberries

Gooseberry Preserve (page 13)

strawberry jelly/jello

200 g/1 1/2 cups strawberries

100 g/1/3 cup strawberry sugar-free jam/jelly (I use St. Dalfour)

2 leaves grass-fed gelatine

custard

150 g/1 cup coconut cream (the solidified coconut from a can of coconut milk or cream, see Note, page 15)

30 g/1 1/2 tablespoons honey

3/4 teaspoon vanilla bean paste (or seeds from 1 vanilla pod/bean)

2 egg yolks

a cake pan, greased and lined with baking parchment

MAKES 4

Preheat the oven to 150°C (300°F) Gas 2.

Melt the coconut oil in a saucepan over low heat and set aside to come back to room temperature. In a separate pan, melt the coconut cream over low heat and set aside to cool to room temperature.

In a stand mixer, or using a handheld electric whisk, mix the eggs and palm sugar together so that the mixture doubles in size and is creamy and lighter in colour than when you started. Add the melted coconut cream and vanilla. Whisk lightly to combine the ingredients – you do not need to mix the ingredients much. Sift in the flours and baking powder, add the coconut oil and mix together. Again do not over-mix. Transfer the mixture to the prepared cake pan and bake in the preheated oven for 15–20 minutes, until an inserted skewer comes out clean.

Store the cake for up to 5 days in an airtight container if not using right away.

To make the strawberry jelly/jello, soak the gelatine leaves in water. Blitz the fresh strawberries and jam/jelly in a food processor until smooth. Gently warm the strawberry mixture in a saucepan over medium heat then squeeze the gelatine of any excess liquid and add to the pan. Whisk to combine. Remove the pan from the heat and leave to cool to room temperature, whisking every so often so that the gelatine is evenly distributed.

To make the custard, warm the coconut cream in a saucepan to melt it down a little. Beat together the honey, vanilla and egg yolks in a mixing bowl. Once the cream is warm, but not hot, slowly pour into the yolk mixture while whisking constantly. Pour everything back into the saucepan and whisk over low heat to thicken. Transfer the fillling to a clean bowl. Lay a piece of clingfilm/plastic wrap over the surface to stop a skin forming and put in the fridge for at least 3 hours.

To layer the trifle, start by fitting slices of cake into glasses or serving bowls. Once the strawberry jelly/jello has reached room temperature pour in a layer on top of the cake. Cover with clingfilm/plastic wrap and put in the fridge for a few hours to set.

Add a layer of gooseberry preserve then some fresh berries. Spoon a layer of custard on top and put in the fridge for 20 minutes before serving.

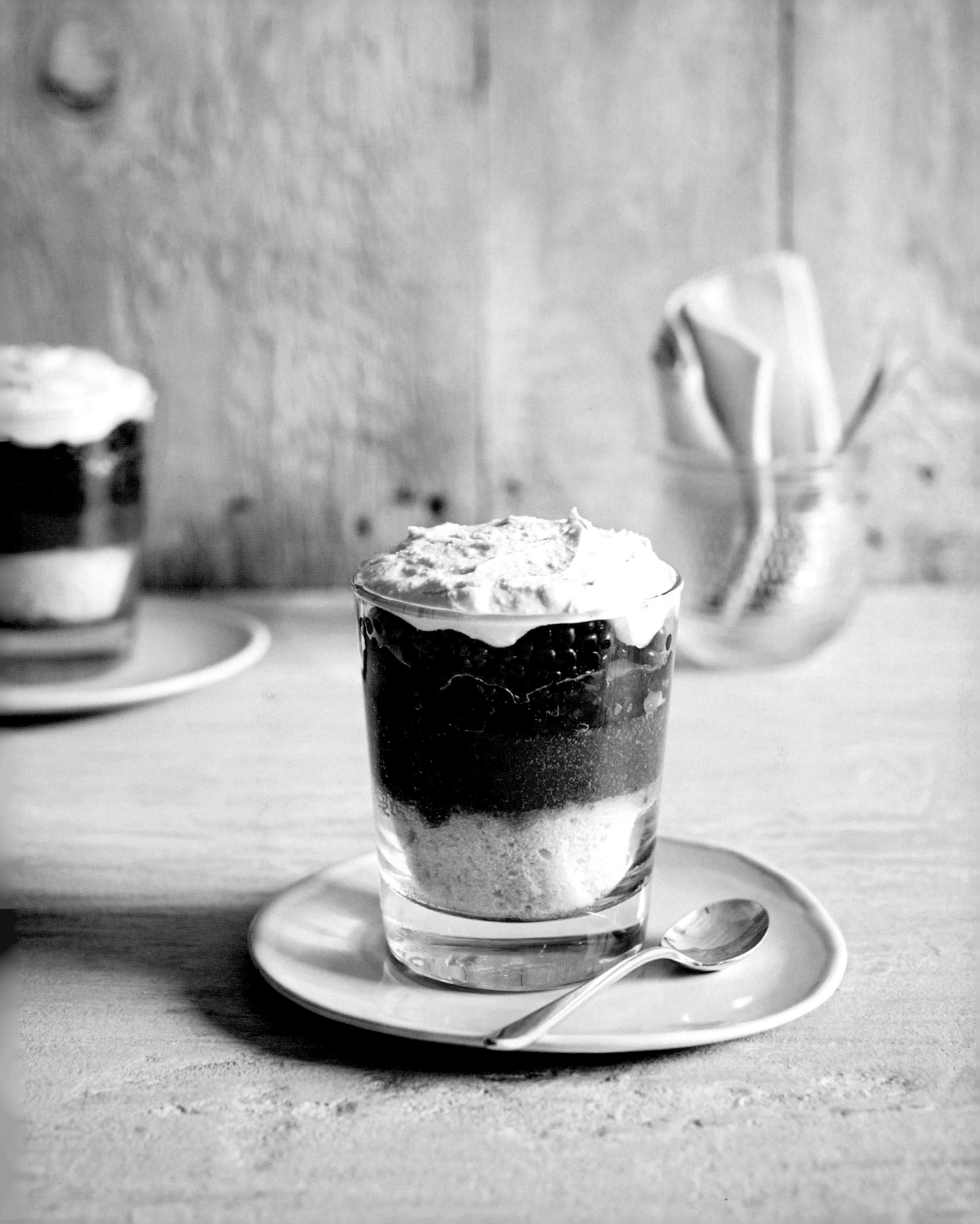

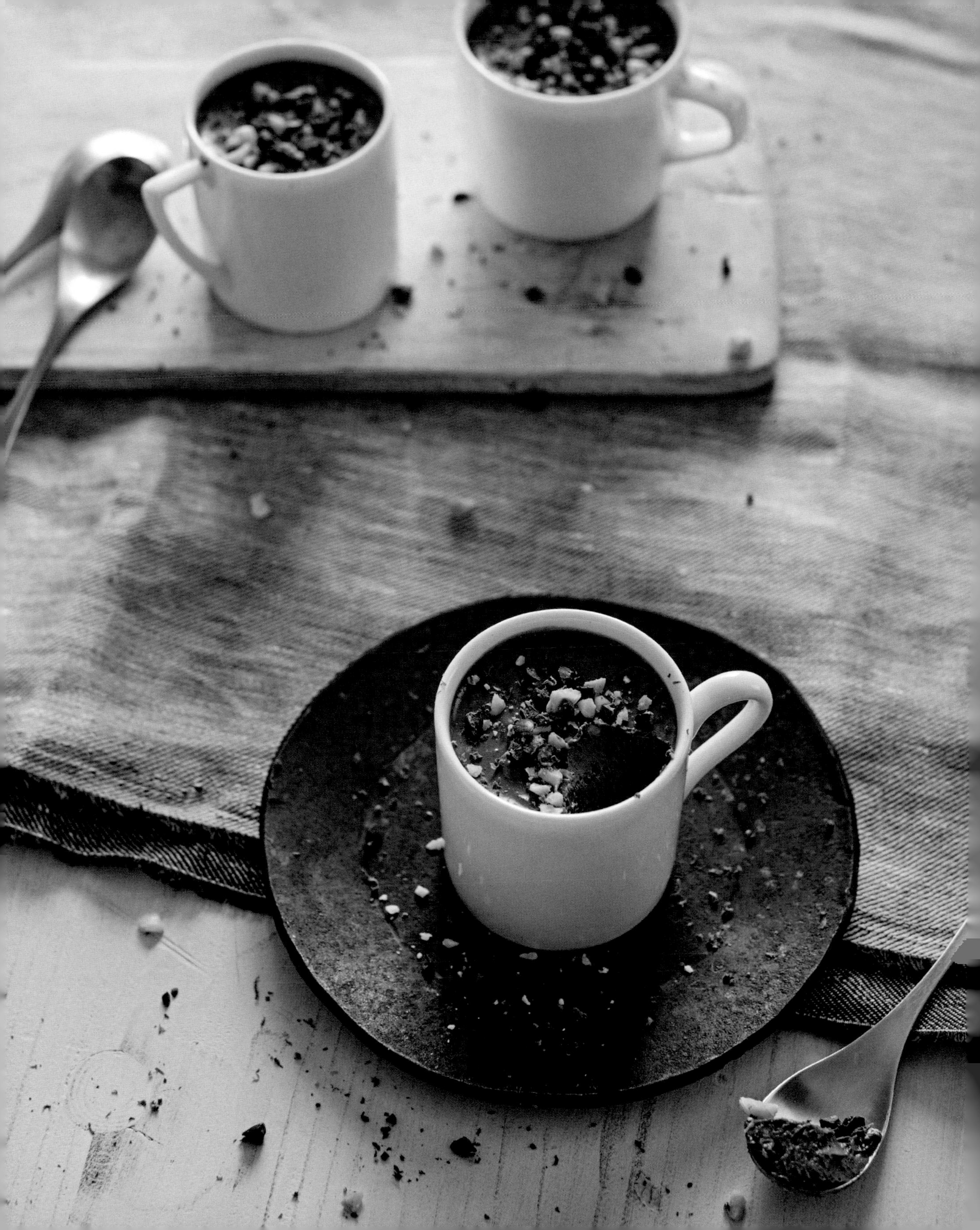

mocha mousse

I like to serve this mousse in coffee cups topped with chopped hazelnuts and ground cacao beans for a bit of fun. You can exchange the coffee and rum (if using) with things like citrus juice and zest, or raspberries if you fancy a change.

300 g/10½ oz. dairy-free dark/bittersweet chocolate

160 ml/⅔ cup coconut cream (the solidified coconut from a can of coconut milk or cream, see Note, page 15)

2 egg yolks

3 egg whites

2 tablespoons palm sugar

2 tablespoons very strong coffee (or coffee extract)

1–2 tablespoons rum (optional)

hazelnuts, toasted to garnish

cacao (or cocoa) nibs, to garnish

SERVES 4

Break the chocolate up into a heatproof bowl. Warm the coconut cream in a saucepan over medium heat and pour over the chocolate to melt. Leave for 5 minutes, stirring occasionally. If the chocolate hasn't completely melted, set the bowl over a pan of simmering water for a moment or two. You want to heat the chocolate as little as possible.

In a separate bowl, whisk together the egg yolks and the palm sugar until light and creamy.

Once the chocolate is cool, but still melted, add this to the egg yolk and sugar mixture with the coffee and rum (if using) and stir until well combined.

In a third bowl, whisk the egg whites using a handheld electric whisk until you have soft peaks. Use a slotted spoon to fold the egg whites into the chocolate mixture.

Spoon the mixture into coffee cups, serving dishes or one large dish. Put in the fridge to set for 2–3 hours.

Top with chopped hazelnuts and cacao nibs to serve.

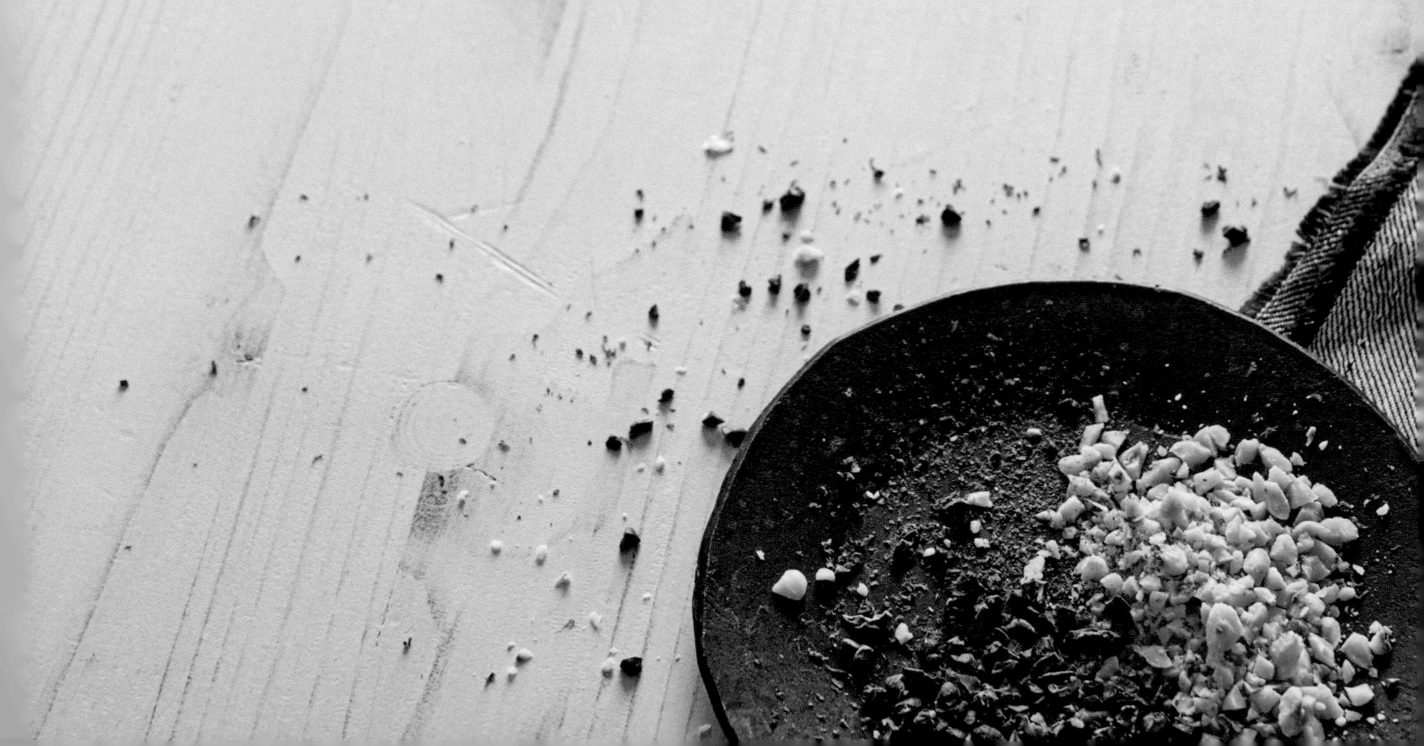

mini carrot cakes

25 g/1 1/2 tablespoons tapioca flour

75 g/3/4 cup ground almonds

1 teaspoon baking powder

1 teaspoon ground cinnamon

1 teaspoon mixed/apple pie spice

a pinch of salt

2 eggs

70 ml/5 tablespoons Sweet Freedom fruit syrup (liquid sweetener)

zest of 1 orange

125 g/1 cup grated carrot

25 g/scant 1/4 cup pecans, roughly chopped

15 g/1/8 cup walnuts, roughly chopped

15 g/2 tablespoons raisins, roughly chopped

citrus frosting

100 g/3/4 cup cashews, soaked in water for 4 hours and rinsed

zest and freshly squeezed juice of 1 lemon

zest and freshly squeezed juice of 1 lime

zest and freshly squeezed juice of 1 orange

30 ml/2 tablespoons honey (or to taste)

a mini loaf pan, greased

a high-powered blender (I use a NutriBullet)

MAKES 8–10

Carrot cake is such a comforting treat, the smells it produces at each cooking stage makes it a very welcoming cake to anyone who might be visiting you. Plus with all that carrot in it, it's practically one of your five-a-day!

Preheat the oven to 160°C (325°F) Gas 3.

Mix together the dry ingredients in a large mixing bowl.

In a separate bowl, whisk together the eggs, fruit syrup and orange zest until light and voluminous.

Whisk the wet mixture into the dry ingredients. Then mix in the grated carrot, nuts and raisins.

Evenly fill the mini loaf pan holes and bake in the preheated oven for 15 minutes. The cakes should be well-risen and springy.

Meanwhile, prepare the citrus frosting. In a high-powdered blender, blitz all the ingredients until smooth and creamy. Taste and add more honey if desired, then set aside.

Remove the cakes from the pan and cool on a wire rack.

Once completely cold, spread with citrus frosting and serve.

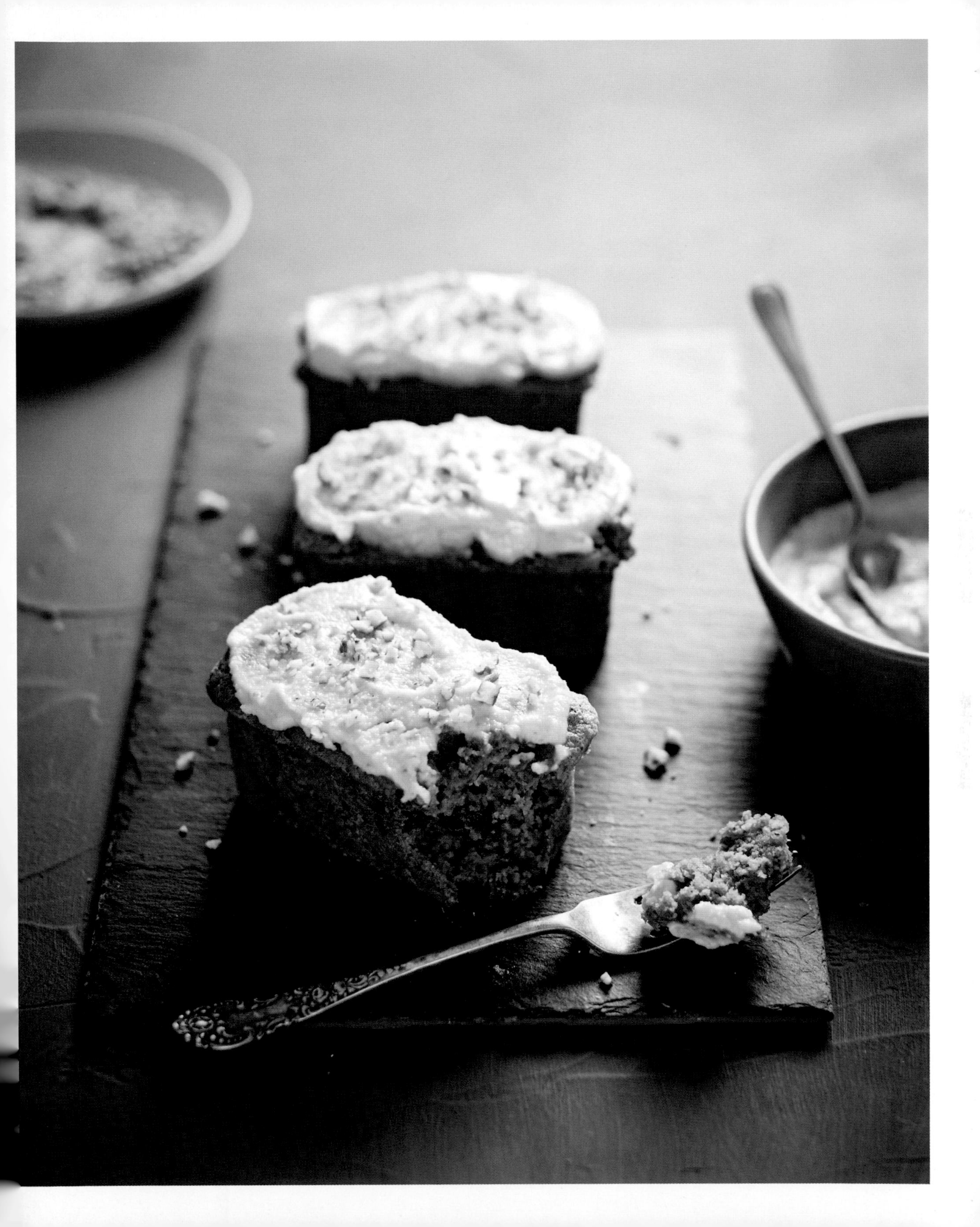

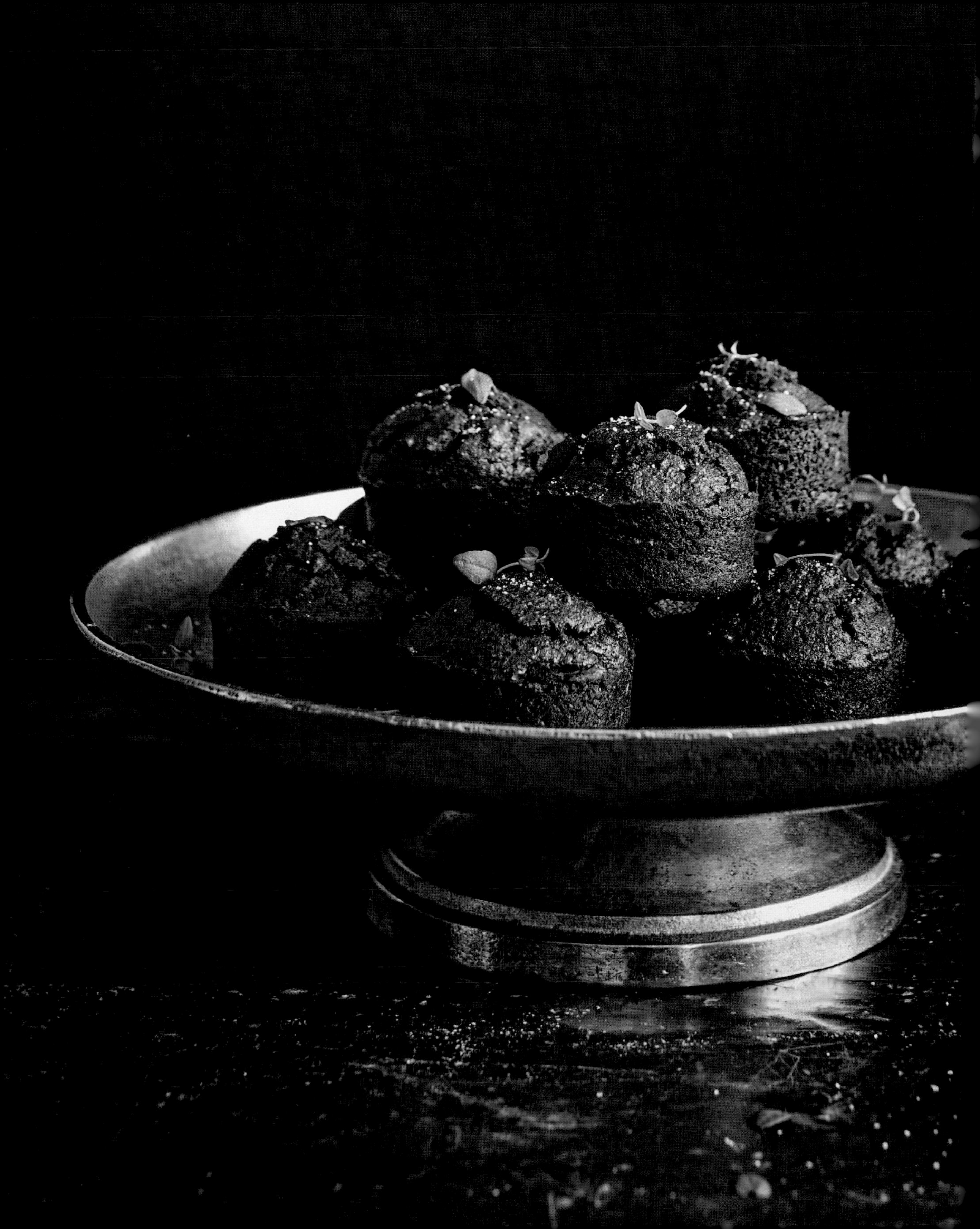

cinnamon and thyme chocolate cupcakes

These are perfect served straight from the oven when they are still warm. Xylitol is a natural sweetener and when I feel like sugar is just not on the agenda it is my go-to alternative. Rich chocolate is lightly spiced with cinnamon and thyme for a deliciously indulgent treat.

140 g/scant 1 1/2 cups ground almonds

80 g/heaped 1/2 cup arrowroot

2 teaspoons baking powder

a pinch of salt

80 g/2/3 cup xylitol

40 g/scant 1/2 cup cocoa (or cacao) powder

4 teaspoons chopped fresh thyme, plus extra to decorate

3 teaspoons ground cinnamon

75 g/4 1/2 tablespoons coconut butter, melted and cooled

4 1/2 tablespoons light olive oil

1 teaspoon vanilla bean paste

4 eggs

extra virgin olive oil, to drizzle

pink Himalayan salt, to sprinkle

a muffin pan, greased and dusted with cocoa (or cacao) powder

MAKES 12

Preheat the oven to 170°C (325°F) Gas 3.

Sift together the dry ingredients, herbs and spices. Any remaining lumps in the sieve/strainer can be put in the mixture.

In a separate bowl, whisk together the coconut butter, oil, vanilla and eggs. Whisk this into the dry mixture.

Divide evenly between the muffin pan holes and bake in the preheated oven for 15–20 minutes or until risen and springy, with a slightly cracked top.

Drizzle with a tiny bit of oil, extra virgin olive oil if you have it, and the tiniest sprinkle of pink Himalayan salt and thyme leaves if desired.

mini lemon and raspberry cakes with lemon curd frosting

The lemon and white chocolate curd frosting here was originally the filling for a lemon tart I made for my first ever Paleo pop-up event. The cakes work well naked (without the frosting) but I think it adds something a little extra. You can try this method with a mixture of citrus fruits if lemon isn't your thing.

3 lemons

6 eggs

150 g/generous 1/2 cup honey

250 g/2 1/2 cups ground almonds

1 teaspoon baking powder

1–2 handfuls of fresh or frozen raspberries

freeze-dried raspberries, to decorate

lemon curd frosting

zest and freshly squeezed juice of 4 lemons

200 g/scant 3/4 cup honey

5 eggs plus 1 egg yolk

150 g/3/4 cup cacao butter (the flavour will differ depending on the brand – I use Choc Chick), roughly chopped

white cacao shards

50 g/3 1/2 tablespoons cacao butter

a squeeze of honey

freeze dried berries

a muffin pan lined with paper cases

MAKES 12

Put the lemons in a large saucepan and cover with water. Set over medium heat and bring to the boil. Continue to boil until soft (this can take 1–2 hours). Once cooked drain the lemons and leave to cool.

Meanwhile, prepare the lemon curd frosting. Put the lemon zest and juice with the honey in a medium saucepan and set over low–medium heat. Whisk to combine and when the honey is dissolved remove from the heat. In a mixing bowl, whisk the eggs and extra egg yolk. While whisking, slowly start to pour in the lemon and honey mixture. It's really important that your juice is warm and not hot as it could scramble the eggs as you work. Return the mixture back to the saucepan and set over low heat. Add the chopped cacao butter. Stir constantly with a whisk then use a spoon or rubber spatula. Be patient and keep the heat low. The mixture will start to thicken – you are looking for a consistency of thick custard and it should coat the back of spoon nicely. Transfer to a bowl to cool, cover the surface with a layer of clingfilm/plastic wrap to stop a film forming and put in the fridge for at least 4 hours to set. I like to make this a day or two before serving as it helps the flavours to develop.

Preheat the oven to 170°C (325°F) Gas 3.

Cut the boiled lemons in half and remove any pips. Blend to a pulp in a food processor and transfer to a large mixing bowl. In a separate bowl, whisk the eggs to get air into them, then mix in the honey, ground almonds, baking powder and lemon. Fold in the fresh or frozen raspberries and divide the mixture between the paper cases. Bake in the preheated oven for 20 minutes. If the cakes are colouring too fast turn down the heat or cover with foil. Test the cakes are cooked with metal skewer and bake for longer if needed. Remove from the oven and cool on a wire rack.

To make the white cacao shards, melt the cacao butter and honey in a heatproof bowl suspended over a pan of barely simmering water. Whisk to combine then pour a thin layer onto a sheet of baking parchment. Sprinkle with freeze-dried raspberries and put in the fridge to set for 2–3 hours.

Once the cakes are cool, spread with the frosting and sprinkle with freeze-dried raspberries. Break up the cacao shards and poke a piece into each cake.

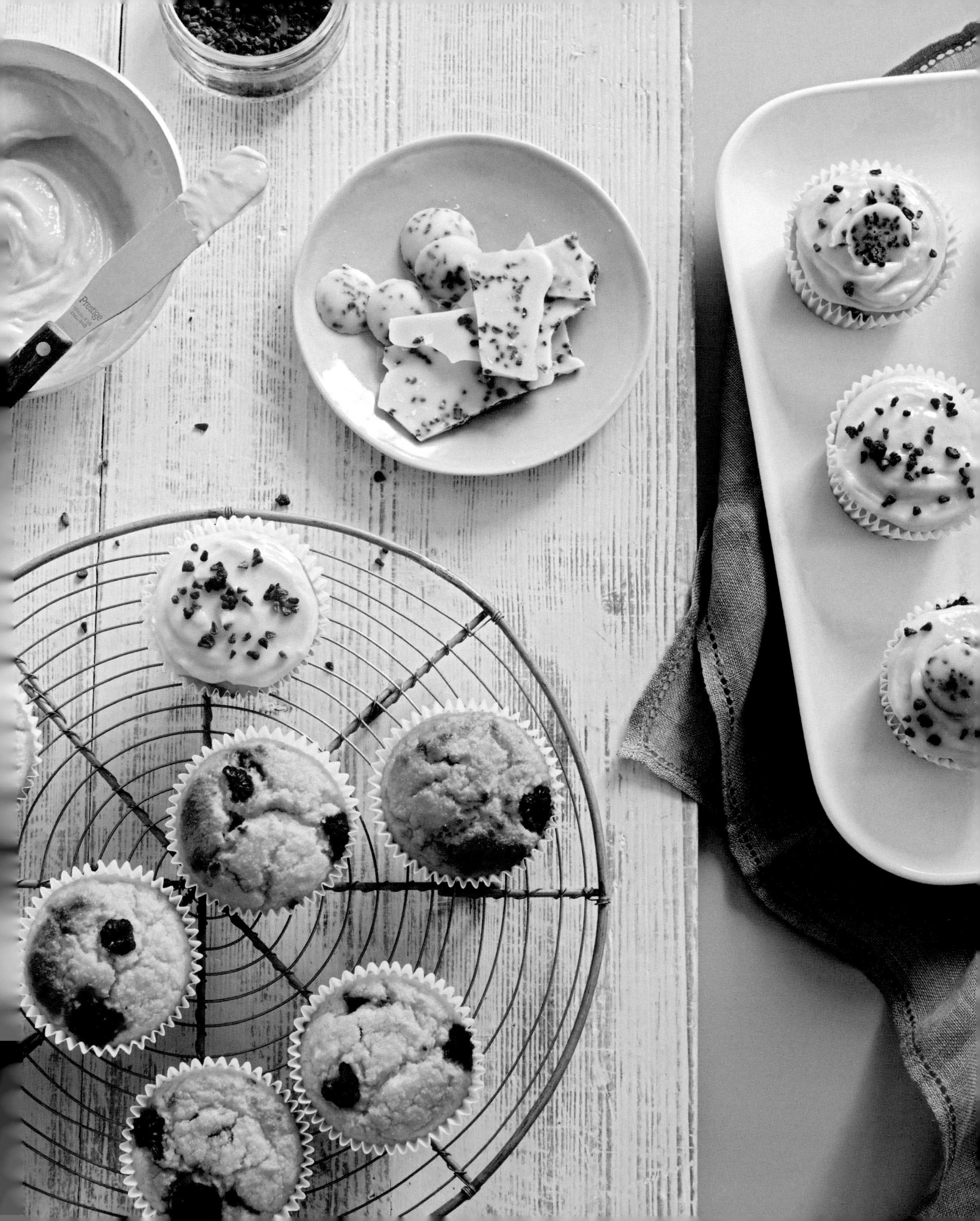
Prestige

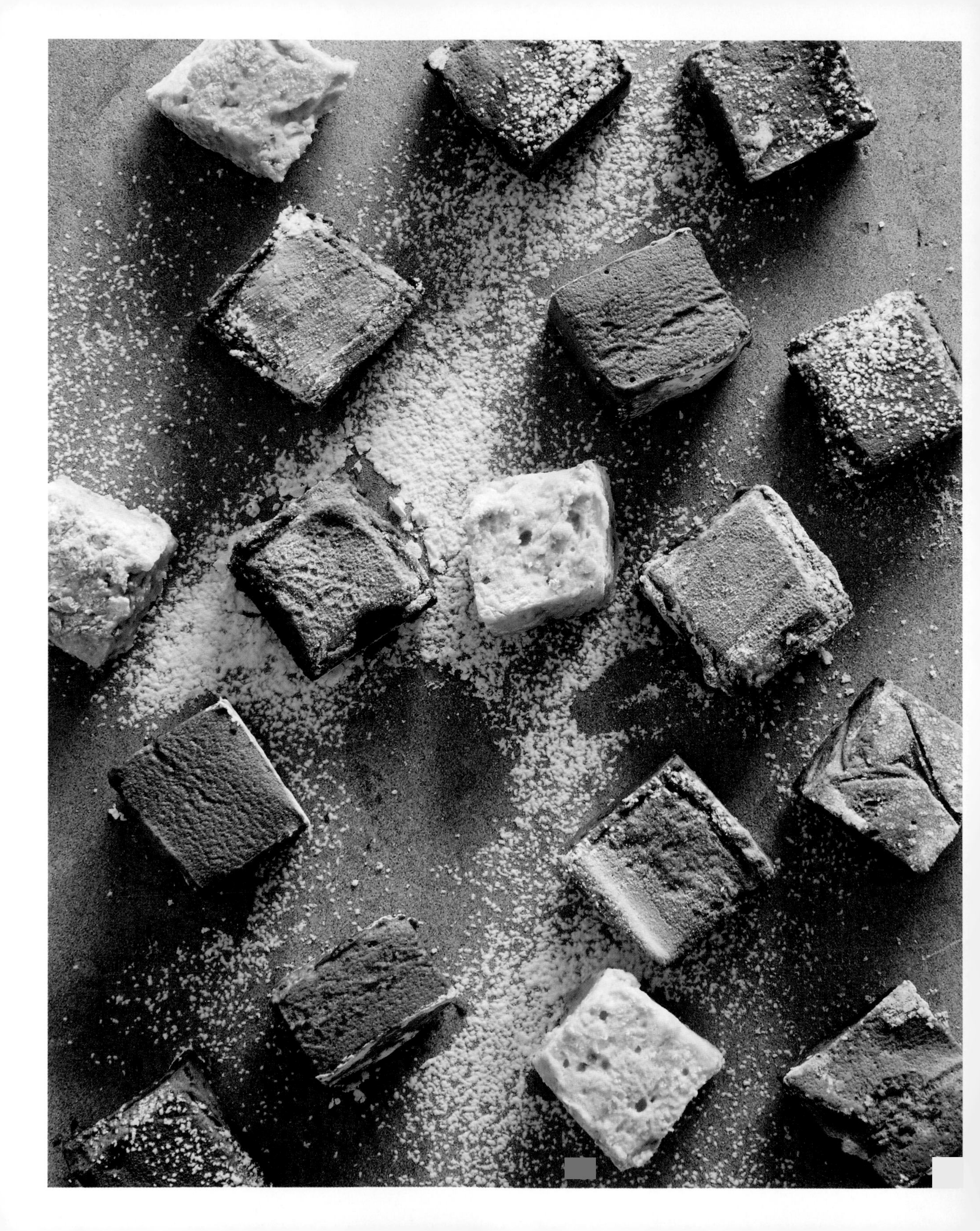

marshmallows

Marshmallows take me back to my childhood. I'm a sucker for colour in my food so I just had to make colourful marshmallows like those I had as a little girl! I advise using a stand mixer because the mixture takes time to come together. Coat the marshmallows in freeze-dried fruits, cocoa powder or ground nuts for a bit of fun.

2 tablespoons grass-fed gelatine (such as Great Lakes)

1 egg white

1 teaspoon pure vanilla extract

arrowroot, to dust

blueberry and juniper

1/2 tablespoon juniper berries

150 ml/2/3 cup blueberry juice (I use Biona Organic)

90 ml/6 tablespoons honey

160 ml/2/3 cup Sweet Freedom fruit syrup (liquid sweetener)

beetroot/beet and cherry

130 ml/1/2 cup honey

70 ml/1/3 cup cherry juice (I use Biona Organic)

2 tablespoons fresh beetroot/beet juice, plus cherry juice to make up to 150 ml/2/3 cup

apricot and honey

130 g/scant 1 cup dried apricots

115 ml/scant 1/2 cup honey

a deep baking pan, oiled and lined with two layers of clingfilm/plastic wrap (lightly oil the clingfilm/plastic wrap)

EACH MAKES ABOUT 30

For blueberry and juniper marshmallows, bring a saucepan filled with 200 ml/3/4 cup of water to a gentle simmer over medium heat. Add the juniper berries, cover with a lid and simmer for 10–20 minutes until the berries soften and begin to break down. Strain the water into a jug/pitcher and set aside.

In a large mixing bowl, use a fork to whisk the blueberry juice with the gelatine. Set aside. Put the egg white into the bowl of a stand mixer.

Warm the honey and fruit syrup with 130 ml/1/2 cup of juniper water in a saucepan over medium heat. Bring to a boil until it reaches 125°C (250°F). Just before the liquid reaches temperature, whisk the egg white to soft peaks.

Quickly but carefully add the liquid to the blueberry and gelatine mixture, then slowly pour this into the egg white with the mixer on. Whisk at full speed until the mixture becomes glossy, light and doubled in volume – this will take about 8 minutes. Add the vanilla extract, continue to whisk for 2 minutes then stop.

Pour the mixture into the prepared baking pan and smooth out the top. Put in the fridge for at least 3 hours to set.

Lift the marshmallow from the pan using the clingfilm/plastic wrap. Carefully grease a sharp knife with a light flavourless oil and use to cut into squares.

Dust the cut marshmallows in arrowroot to coat and seal them so they are not too sticky to pick up. Pat off any excess and enjoy.

For beetroot/beet and cherry marshmallows, put the honey and cherry juice in a large saucepan over medium heat. Bring to 125°C (250°F). In a large mixing bowl, use a fork to whisk the gelatine powder with the beetroot/beet juice instead of blueberry juice. Put the egg white into the bowl of a stand mixer, add the warmed honey and cherry juice and follow the instructions as above.

For apricot and honey marshmallows, put the dried apricots in a saucepan with enough water to cover and a lid. Simmer over medium heat until the apricots soften. Strain, discarding the water, then push through a fine-mesh sieve/strainer using the back of a spoon to make a purée. Any remaining apricot pulp can be added to the purée and mixed through. In the bowl of the stand mixer, use a fork to whisk together the gelatine and 75 ml/5 tablespoons of water. In a saucepan, bring the honey and 110 ml/scant 1/2 cup of water to 125°C (250°F). With the motor running, slowly pour the hot honeyed water into the mixer. Whisk on a high speed for 8 minutes, then follow the instructions as above.

peach slice with cognac ice cream

I originally wrote this recipe when I was working at Pure Taste. I love the flavour combinations of the soft, sweet peach and the sharp and smooth Cognac. I sometimes add fresh raspberries for a bit of extra colour and flavour.

2 peaches, halved, stoned/pitted and cut into slices

coconut oil, for frying

100 g/¼ cup sliced canned peaches, blitzed to a purée

140 ml/generous ½ cup coconut cream (the solidified coconut from a can of coconut milk or cream, see Note, page 15)

1 egg

30 ml/2 tablespoons honey

20 g/1½ tablespoons coconut flour

100 g/1 cup ground almonds

½ teaspoon baking powder

flaked/slivered almonds, to sprinkle

Cognac Ice Cream (page 140), to serve

a high-powered blender (I use a NutriBullet)

a 23-cm/9-inch square cake pan, greased and lined with baking parchment

SERVES 10

Preheat the oven to 160°C (325°F) Gas 3.

Put a small amount of coconut oil in a non-stick frying pan/skillet over medium heat. Fry the peach slices in the oil and caramelize on each side. Remove from the pan and set aside until ready to serve.

Put the canned peaches in the blender and blitz to a purée. Add the coconut cream, egg and honey, and blitz again until smooth.

Add the coconut flour, ground almonds and baking powder. Blitz again until well combined.

Pour into the prepared cake pan, top with the caramelized peach slices in rows and sprinkle with flaked/slivered almonds.

Bake in the preheated oven for 25–30 minutes until golden. Leave to cool on a wire rack for 15 minutes, then put in fridge until it is completely cold.

Once cold, lift out of the pan and cut into 10 even slices.

Serve with the Cognac ice cream.

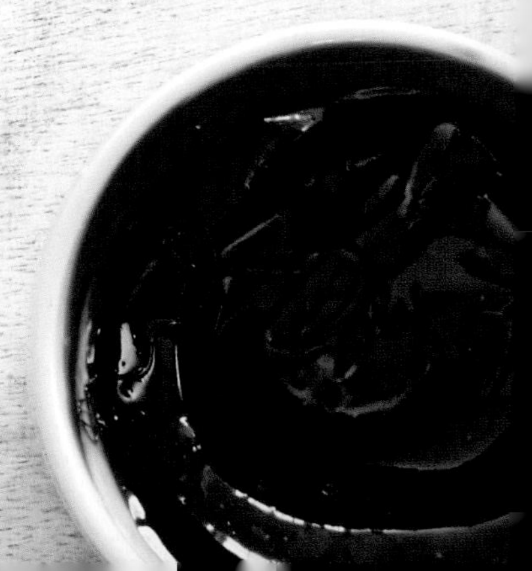

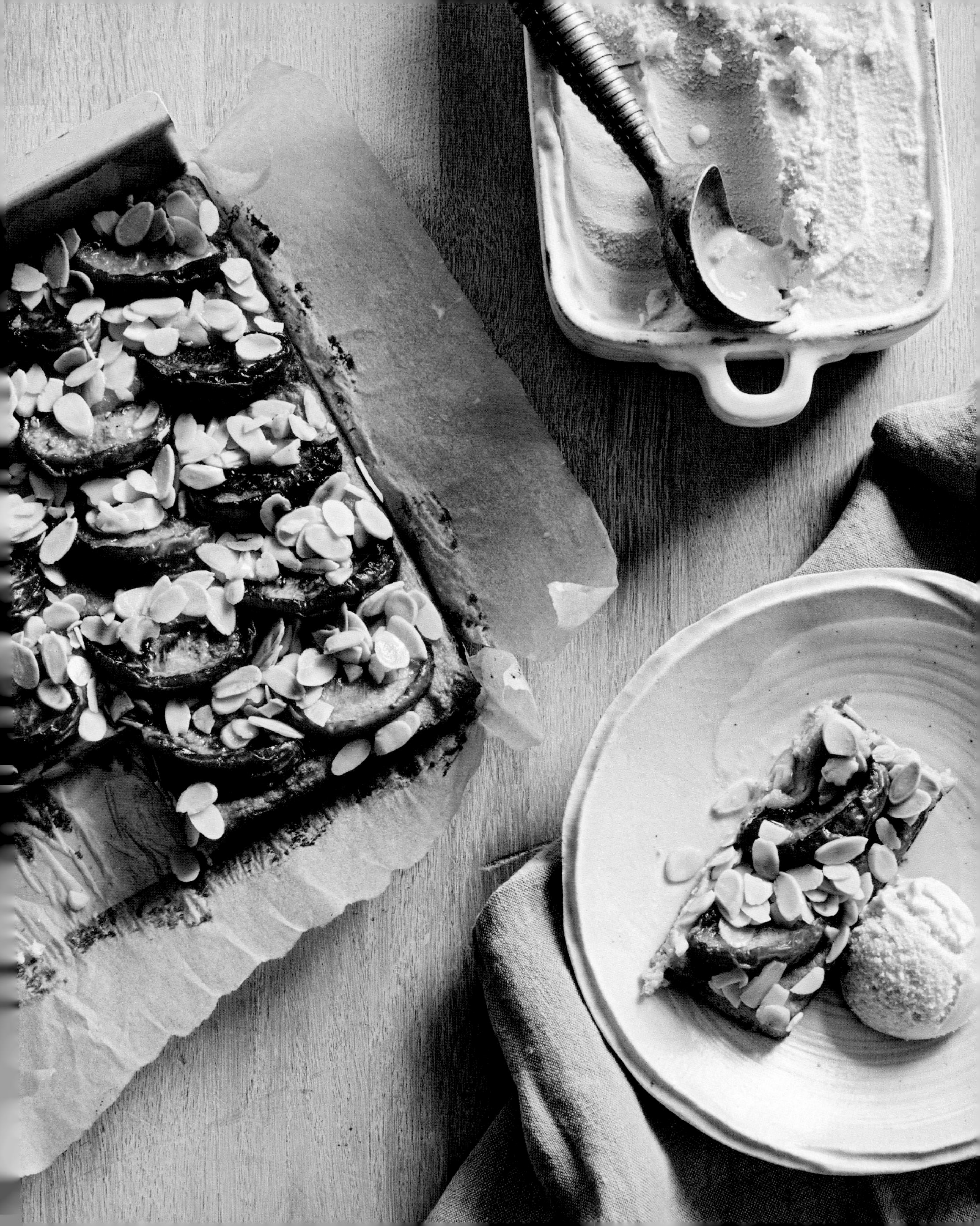

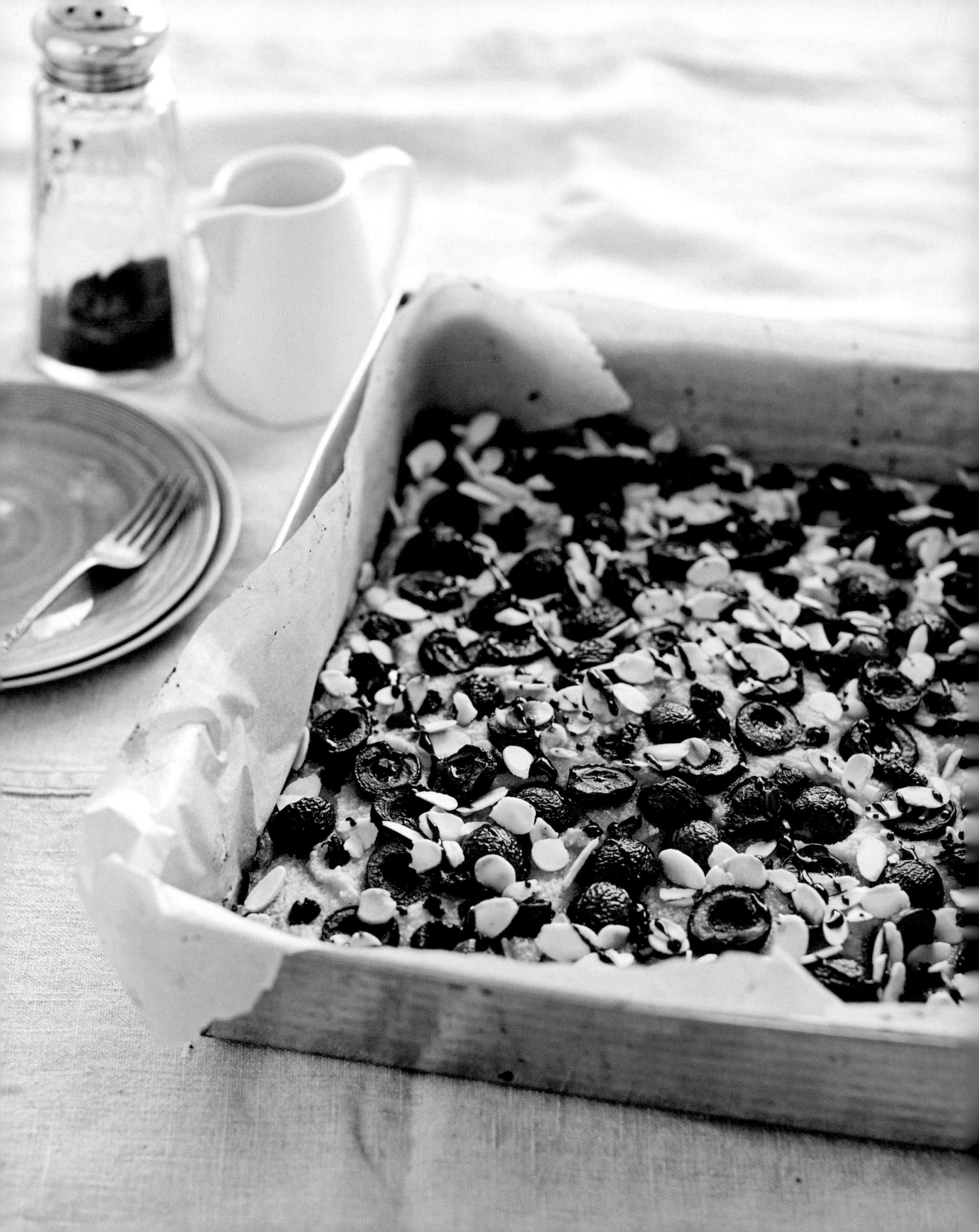

frangipane tray bake

Enjoy a slice of this tray bake as a dessert or with a selection of other afternoon tea treats. I like to serve it with the spiced crème anglaise on page 132, but infuse it with cardamom pods instead of cinnamon. Try this recipe using different fruit toppings – I love a rhubarb frangipane tray bake as a the next best choice following cherry.

230 g/½ lb. whole cherries, halved and stoned/pitted

50 g/⅓ cup sour/tart cherries, roughly chopped (I use Biona Organic)

flaked/slivered almonds, to sprinkle

unsweetened cocoa powder to dust (optional)

cherry syrup

600 ml/2½ cups cherry juice (I use Biona Organic)

honey (or maple syrup), to taste (optional)

pastry

80 g/⅔ cup arrowroot

185 g/generous 1¾ cups almond flour

80 g/5½ tablespoons coconut butter

1 egg, plus 1 beaten egg, for brushing

almond frangipane

270 g/2¾ cups ground almonds

150 g/generous ½ cup honey

75 ml/⅓ cup hemp milk

3 tablespoons coconut flour

seeds from 1 vanilla pod/bean

2½ teaspoons pure almond extract

3 eggs

a 30 x 25-cm/12 x 10-inch baking pan, greased and lined with baking parchment

SERVES 8–10

To make a cherry syrup, pour the cherry juice into a saucepan and simmer over medium heat until the juice reduces down and is thick and glossy. You can add a little honey or maple syrup if the result is too sharp for your taste. Set aside until ready to serve.

Preheat the oven to 180°C (350°F) Gas 4.

To make the pastry, mix together the arrowroot and almond flour in a large mixing bowl and rub in the coconut butter.

In a separate bowl, beat the egg and 3–4 tablespoons of water together and add this to the flour mixture. Mix together and form a dough. Roll out between two pieces of baking parchment to the size of the baking pan and transfer to the pan.

Brush the pastry with the beaten egg and bake in the preheated oven for 10 minutes, or until golden. Keep the oven on.

To make the almond frangipane, mix all of the ingredients together.

Spread the almond frangipane evenly across baked pastry base and top with the halved and sour/tart cherries. Sprinkle with flaked/slivered almonds and bake in the still warm oven for 20–30 minutes until golden.

Drizzle with the reserved cherry syrup and dust with cocoa powder if desired, slice and serve.

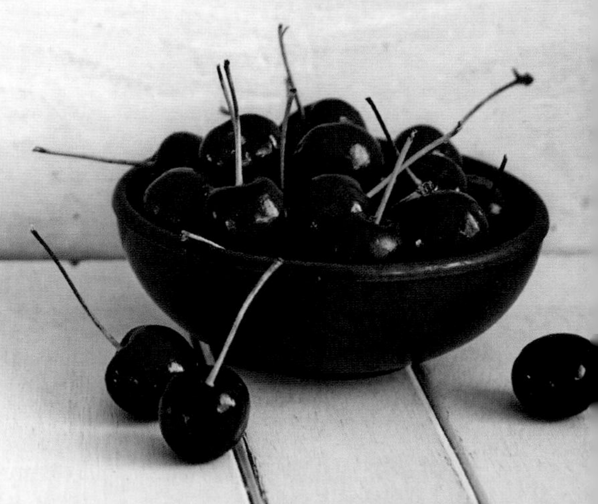

campfire pie

This recipe has been developed from some very fond memories of mine. When I was young, my sisters and I often used to set up a campfire and tents in our garden. We would wrap bananas in foil with chocolate, put them in the fire. Then hunt around for acceptable marshmallow sticks. Marshmallows toasted on an open fire were my all-time favourite treat then and still are now.

25 g/1¾ tablespoons cacao butter

25 g/1 tablespoon plus 1 teaspoon honey

200 g/1½ cups whole almonds, ground

chocolate and banana filling

100 g/⅓ cup honey

30 g/⅓ cup cacao (or cocoa) powder

30 g/2 tablespoons coconut oil

30 ml/2 tablespoons coconut milk (I use Koko® Dairy Free)

3–4 bananas (or more if you want!), sliced

marshmallow topping

1 heaped tablespoon grass-fed gelatine (such as Great Lakes)

140 g/½ cup honey

1 teaspoon pure vanilla extract

a 20-cm/8-inch fluted cake pan, greased

a chef's blow torch (optional)

SERVES 8–10

Preheat the oven to 140°C (275°F) Gas 1.

To create a base, melt the cacao butter and honey together in a saucepan over low heat. Mix in the ground almonds, then press into the bottom and up the sides of the prepared cake pan.

Bake in the preheated oven for 7–10 minutes, or until slightly golden. Don't worry if the pastry still feels soft – the cacao butter solidifies in the fridge later. Set aside to cool.

To make the chocolate banana layer, bring the honey, cocoa powder and coconut oil to a simmer in a saucepan over low–medium heat for a minute or two. Stir well – the mixture should become glossy and look a little like caramel. Pour in the coconut milk and stir again.

Pour on top of the almond base in the cake pan and put in the fridge to set.

To make the marshmallow topping, dissolve the gelatine in 75 ml/5 tablespoons of water in a stand mixer.

Put the honey and 170 ml/¾ cup of water into a saucepan and bring to a temperature of at least 125°C (250°F).

Turn on the stand mixer and slowly pour the honeyed water into the gelatine. Whisk on high for 10–15 minutes until the mixture becomes white, light and able to hold its peaks. Add the vanilla and just whisk in.

You will only need about half of this mixture for the pie itself – the rest can be put in the fridge to set, following the instruction on page 123.

Lay banana slices over the set chocolate layer and spread the marshmallow topping over the top. Make sure there is texture to the marshmallow topping by swirling it with a spoon or spatula. Put in the fridge to set.

When ready to serve, toast with a chef's blow torch or under a hot grill/broiler.

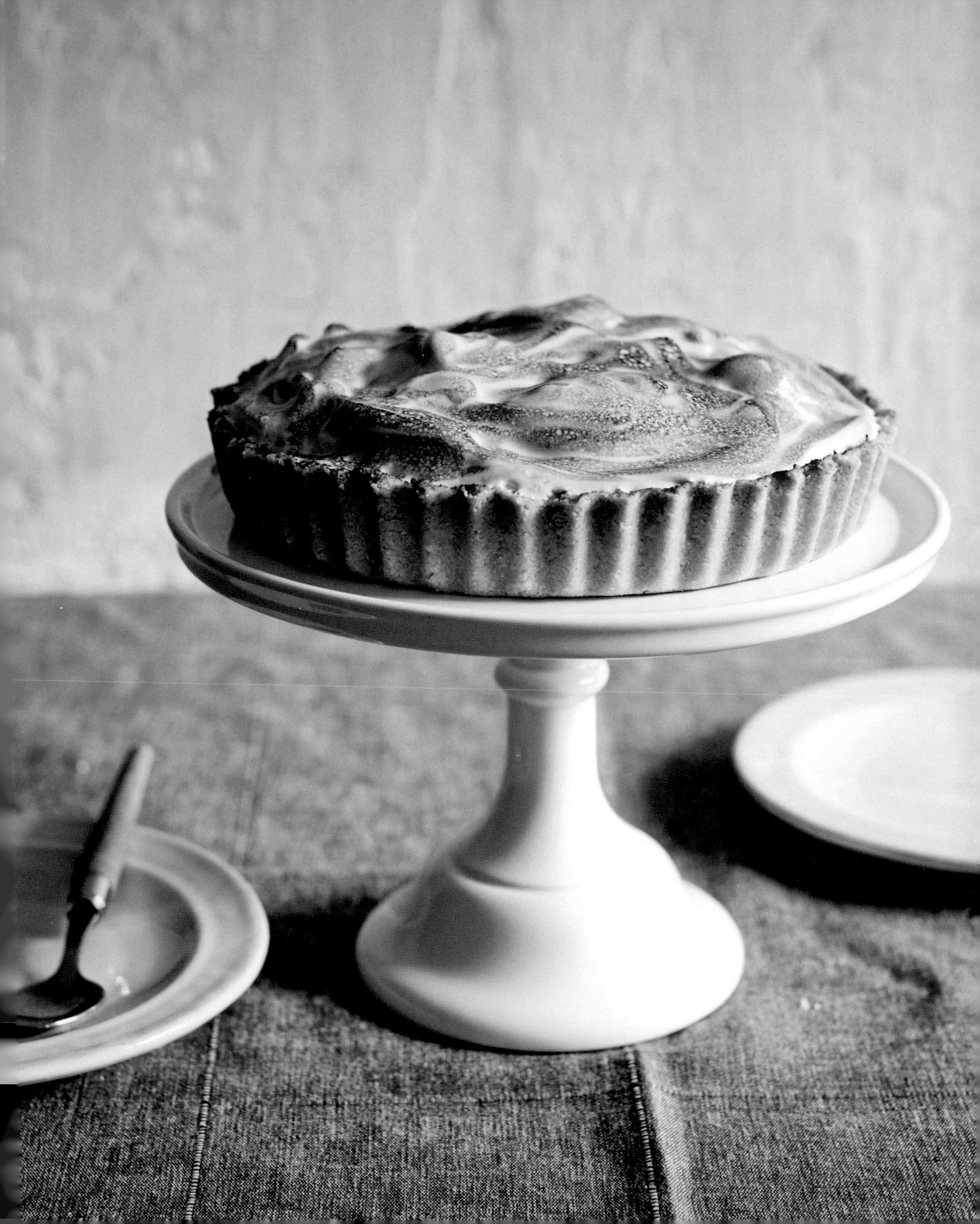

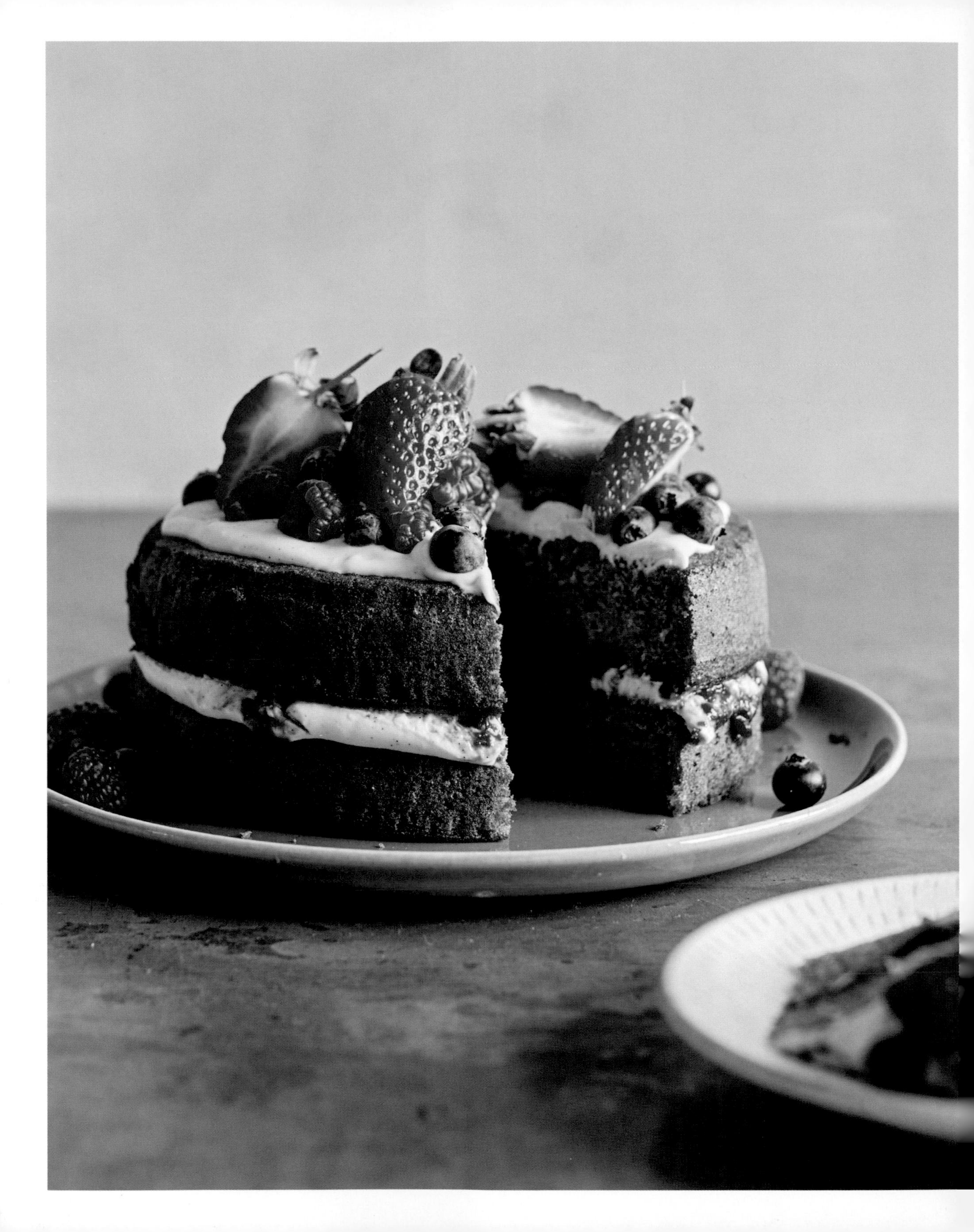

victoria sponge

When I wrote this recipe I wanted to come up with a nut-free Paleo cake as nut flours seem to be the biggest replacement for wheat flours and can be hard to digest. I always get a little nervous sharing my Paleo creations with foodie friends but fellow author Milli Taylor's seal of approval meant I just had to share it with you.

150 g/1 cup coconut oil

150 ml/1 cup coconut cream (the solidified coconut from a can of coconut milk or cream, see Note, page 15)

6 eggs

200 g/7 oz. palm sugar

1 teaspoon pure vanilla extract

70 g/½ cup coconut flour

40 g/¼ cup tapioca flour

2 teaspoons baking powder

Summer Berry Preserve (page 12, or use St. Dalfour), to fill

fresh summer berries, larger ones sliced to serve

cream filling

150 g/1 cup coconut cream (the solidified coconut from a can of coconut milk or cream, see Note, page 15)

30 g/1½ tablespoons honey

¾ teaspoon vanilla bean paste (or seeds from 1 vanilla pod/bean)

2 egg yolks

2 x 20-cm/8-inch round cake pans, greased

SERVES 10–12

Preheat the oven to 150°C (300°F) Gas 2.

Melt the coconut oil in a saucepan over low heat and set aside to come back to room temperature. In a separate pan, melt the coconut cream and set aside to cool to room temperature.

In a stand mixer or using a handheld electric whisk, whisk the eggs and palm sugar together so that the mixture doubles in size and is creamy and lighter in colour than when you started. Add the melted coconut cream and vanilla. Whisk lightly to combine the ingredients – you do not need to mix the ingredients much. Sift in the flours and baking powder, add the coconut oil and mix together. Again do not over-mix.

Divide the mixture between the cake pans and bake in the preheated oven for 15–20 minutes. You may need to bake one at a time so that each cake cooks evenly in the oven.

Meanwhile, prepare the cream filling. Warm the coconut cream in a saucepan to melt it down a little. Beat together the honey, vanilla and egg yolks in a mixing bowl. Once the cream is warm, but not hot, slowly pour into the yolk mixture while whisking constantly. Pour everything back into the saucepan and whisk over low heat to thicken. Transfer the filllling to a clean bowl. Lay a piece of clingfilm/plastic wrap over the surface to stop a skin forming and put in the fridge for at least 3 hours before use so that it solidifies.

Remove the cakes from the oven and put on a wire rack to cool slightly before turning out. Leave on the wire rack to cool completely before filling the cakes.

Spread the cakes with the cream filling and dollop one with summer berry preserve. Top with the second cake and fresh berries. Remember, like butter cream, coconut cream loosens in heat, so store the cake in the fridge unless you are eating it right away.

pear and fig tart

Another recipe where the fruit can easily be changed depending on what's available or in season – I love using apples and blackberries when autumn/fall is approaching.

250 g/2$^{1}/_{2}$ cups ground almonds

40 g/2$^{1}/_{2}$ tablespoons unscented coconut oil, melted

50 g/2$^{1}/_{2}$ tablespoons pure maple syrup

a pinch of fine sea salt

ground cinnamon, to sprinkle

spiced crème anglaise

250 ml/1$^{3}/_{4}$ cup coconut cream (see Note, page 15)

50 g/2$^{1}/_{2}$ tablespoons pure maple syrup

1–2 teaspoons ground cinnamon

1 teaspoon vanilla bean paste (or seeds from 1 vanilla pod/bean)

3 egg yolks

fruit topping

6 pears, peeled, halved, cored and thinly sliced

3 figs, halved or quartered

a 20-cm/8-inch tart pan, lined with baking parchment

a baking sheet lined with baking parchment

SERVES 12

Preheat the oven to 150°C (300°F) Gas 2.

Mix the ground almonds, coconut oil, maple syrup and salt together in a large mixing bowl with a wooden spoon or spatula.

Press the mixture into and up the sides of the prepared tart pan.

Bake in the preheated oven for 8–10 minutes, or until a nice golden, but not brown colour. Remove from the oven, cool and put in the fridge to set.

To make the spiced crème anglaise, warm the coconut cream in a saucepan over low heat to melt it down. In a separate bowl, beat together the maple syrup, cinnamon, vanilla and egg yolks.

Once the cream is warm, but not hot, slowly pour into the yolk mixture, whisking constantly. Pour the mixture back into the saucepan and whisk over low heat until it thickens. Remove the pan from the heat and pour over the tart base. Return to the fridge until the fruit is ready to go on top.

Reduce the oven to 120°C (250°F) Gas $^{1}/_{2}$.

Lay the pear slices flat on the prepared baking sheet. I thinly slice pears, lift them off the board with a palette knife to transfer to the sheet, then push slightly so they flatten and fan out. Bake in the oven for 5–15 minutes until just coloured – you don't want to overcook the fruit because you still need to be able to pick it up and transfer to the tart.

Once cool, and using the palette knife again, lift up each half-pear and lay around the outside of the tart to form a pear circle. Pile the cut figs in the centre of the tart.

Store in the fridge until ready to enjoy. Sprinkle with ground cinnamon before serving. If the tart sits around a couple of days be wary the base will soften, however it will still be super tasty!

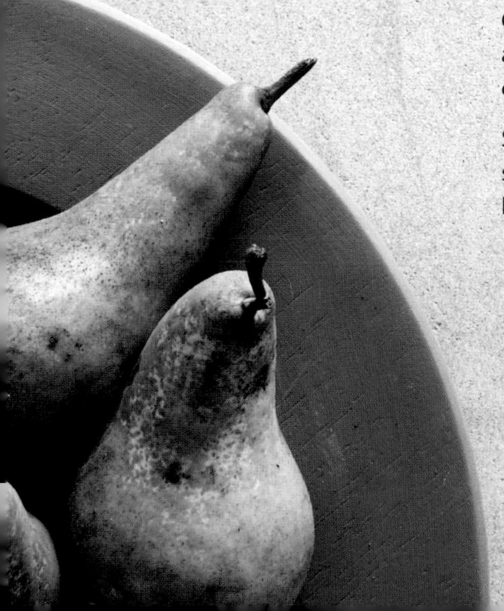

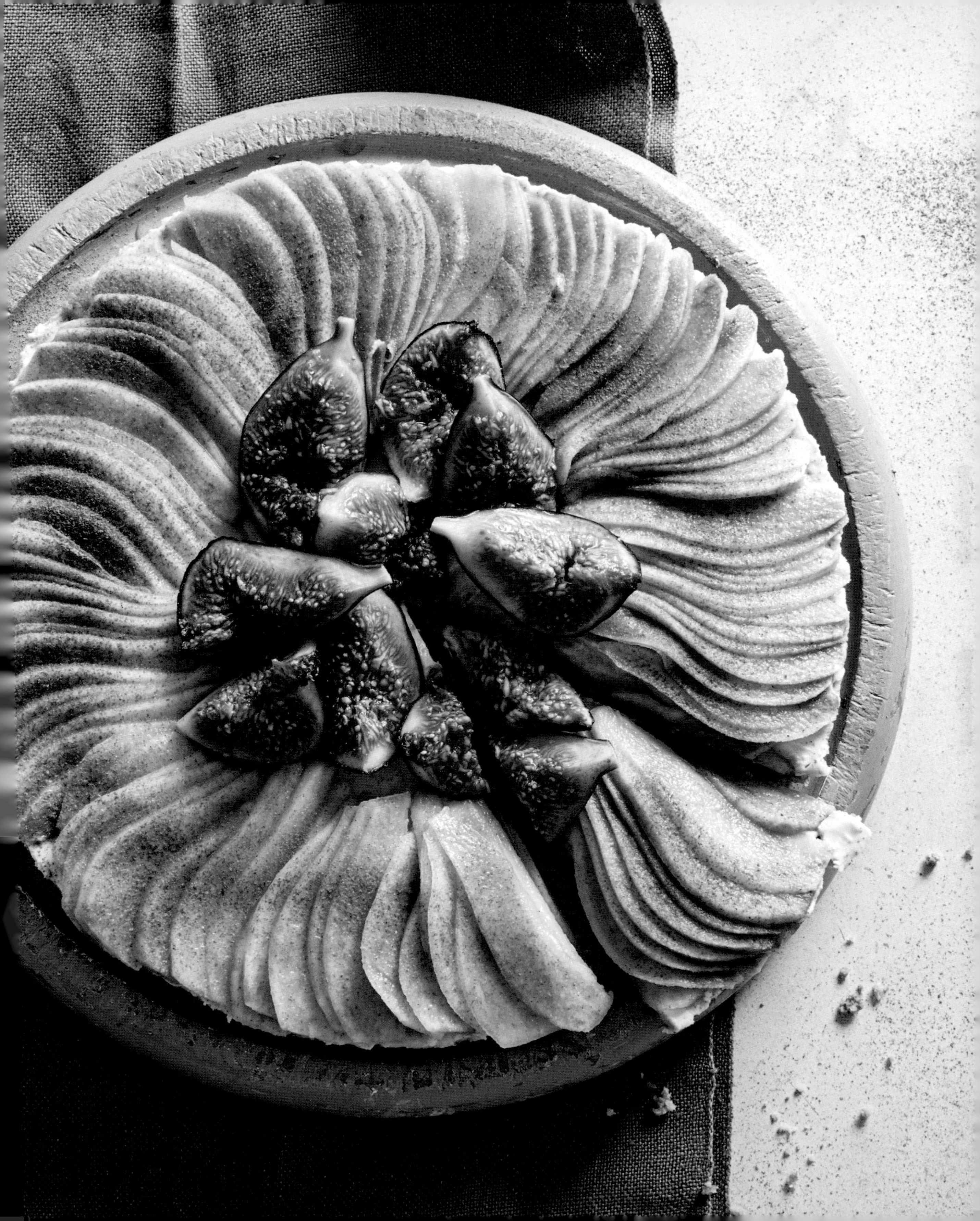

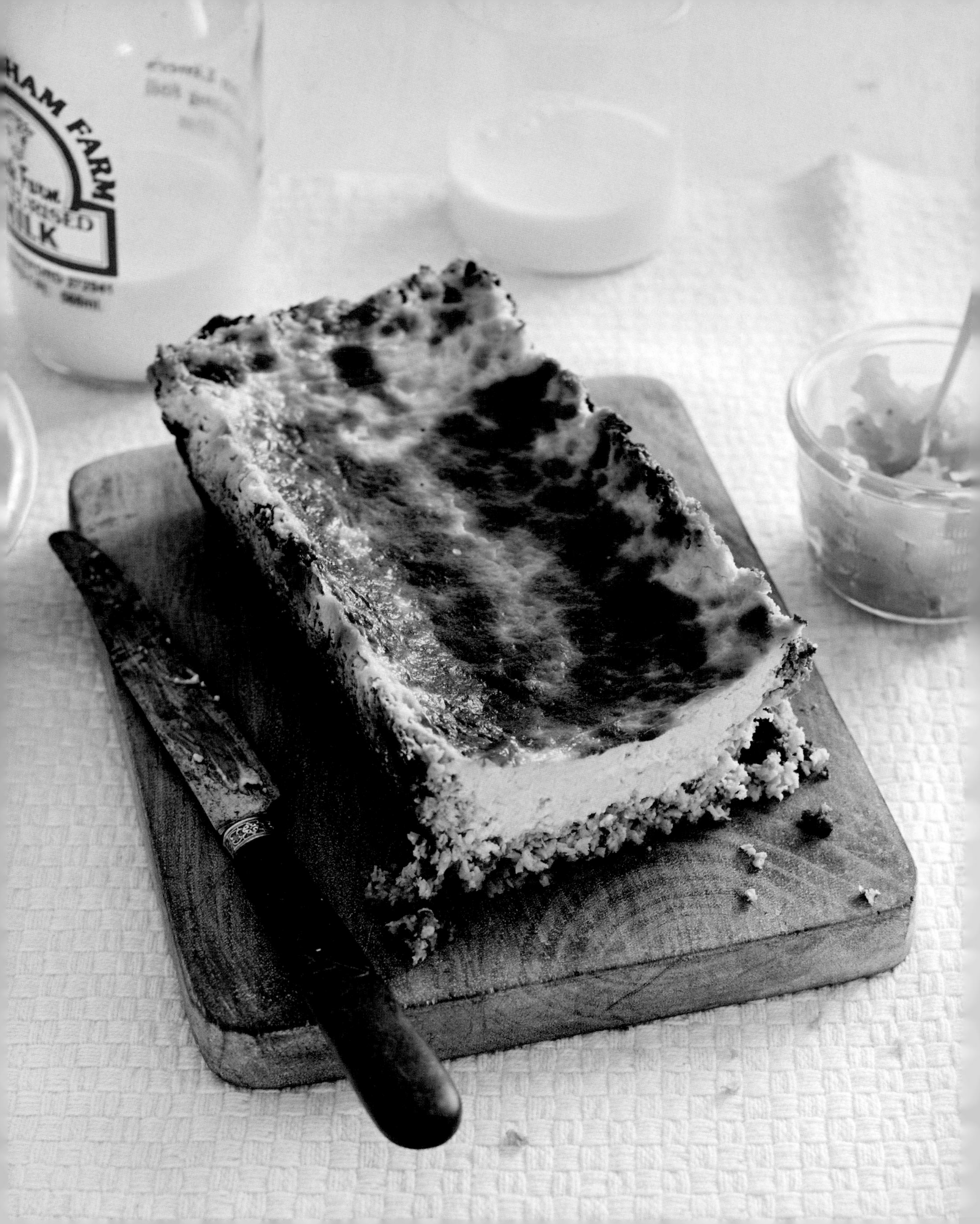
HAM FARM
ILK

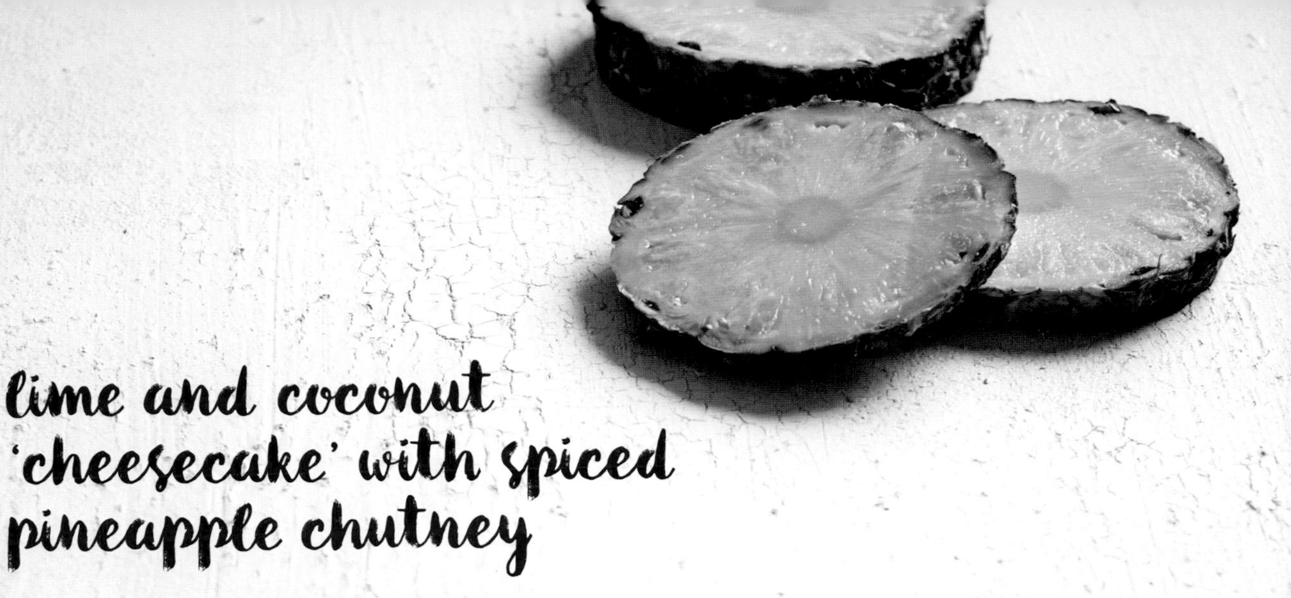

lime and coconut 'cheesecake' with spiced pineapple chutney

The only Paleo 'cheesecakes' I've come across are loaded with nuts, a nutty base with a nut cheese filling. It doesn't always suit me, so this nut-free option is a good one to have in your repertoire.

70 g/2½ oz. pineapple, peeled and diced

2 teaspoons ground ginger

3 dates, soaked in water

175 g/2⅓ cups desiccated/ shredded coconut

coconut oil, for frying

lime and coconut filling

500 ml/2 cups coconut cream

50 g/2½ tablespoons honey

zest and freshly squeezed juice of 5 limes

2 eggs plus 2 egg yolks

spiced pineapple chutney

½ pineapple, peeled and diced

2–3 slivers of fresh ginger

30 g/1¾ tablespoons honey

a rectangular loaf pan, greased and lined with baking parchment

SERVES 8–10

Preheat the oven to 150°C (300°F) Gas 2.

Put a little coconut oil in a frying pan/skillet over medium heat and add the diced pineapple to caramelize.

Transfer to a food processor and add the ground ginger, soaked dates and desiccated/shredded coconut. Blend to combine.

Press the mixture into the base and up the sides of the prepared loaf pan. Bake in the preheated oven for 10–15 minutes, ensuring the coconut doesn't catch.

Remove from the oven and cool on a wire rack. Keep the oven on.

Meanwhile, prepare the lime and coconut filling. Blend all the ingredients in a food processor and pour into the cooled base.

Bake in the still warm oven for 45 minutes, or until cooked – the top will start to colour, which is what you want, however you may need to cover with foil part-way through the bake to avoid it burning. The filling will have a slight wobble when it is ready.

Remove from the oven and leave to cool in the pan on a wire rack. Once cool put in the fridge for at least 1 hour before removing from the pan.

To make the spiced pineapple chutney, put all the ingredients in a saucepan over medium heat. Add just a small amount of water to stop the ingredients from catching on the bottom of the pan and simmer for about 30 minutes until the water has evaporated, leaving a thick sauce over the pineapple.

Serve with the cheesecake.

golden snow dome

This is a great recipe for bringing a bit of colour and excitement to the table at the end of a meal. I know it's quite a long-winded recipe, so don't feel you have to do it as a dome or include every part. For a quicker, easier version, just cook the cake in a regular cake pan and add fresh fruit and coconut ice cream to serve.

150 g/1 1/2 cups ground almonds

25 g/2 tablespoons coconut flour

1 teaspoon baking powder

1 teaspoon ground turmeric

3 eggs

70 g/1/4 cup carob fruit syrup (I use Clarks)

30 g/2 tablespoons coconut oil, melted and cooled plus extra for greasing

a splash of rum (optional)

coconut ice cream

250 ml/1 cup coconut cream

1/2 tablespoon carob fruit syrup

1 tablespoon desiccated/ shredded coconut

to decorate

1 mango, thinly sliced

1 papaya, thinly sliced

desiccated/shredded coconut

a dome cake bowl (or ovenproof bowl), greased

an ice cream maker

SERVES 8–10

Preheat the oven to 170°C (325°F) Gas 3.

Mix together all the dry ingredients in a large mixing bowl.

In a separate bowl, whisk the eggs with the fruit syrup until they start to become lighter and increased in volume, then whisk in the melted oil.

Add the egg mixture to the dry ingredients and mix well. I always use an electric handheld whisk for this. To start with the mix will seem like it will be too wet, but coconut flour is very absorbing so don't worry, it will come together.

You should be able to tease the mixture up the side of the prepared bowl so that you can keep the middle hollow for the ice cream.

Bake in the preheated oven for 15–20 minutes.

Brush with rum (if using) when it comes out of the oven and leave to cool.

To make the coconut ice cream, mix together the ingredients and blend in an ice cream maker, following the manufacturer's instructions.

Spoon the ice cream into the hollow of the cake, cover with foil and put in the freezer for at least 2 hours or until ready to serve.

Remove from the freezer and remove the cake from the bowl – you may need to leave it for 15 minutes before doing this if the cake is stuck in the bowl.

Level off the bottom of the cake if necessary.

Turn upside down on a serving plate and leave until ready to serve. You don't need to worry about the ice cream melting – coconut cream stays set in the fridge. But you want it to be cold enough for your enjoyment and for full golden snow dome effect.

Arrange the sliced fresh mango and papaya around the outside of the dome and sprinkle with desiccated/shredded coconut.

Slice and serve right away.

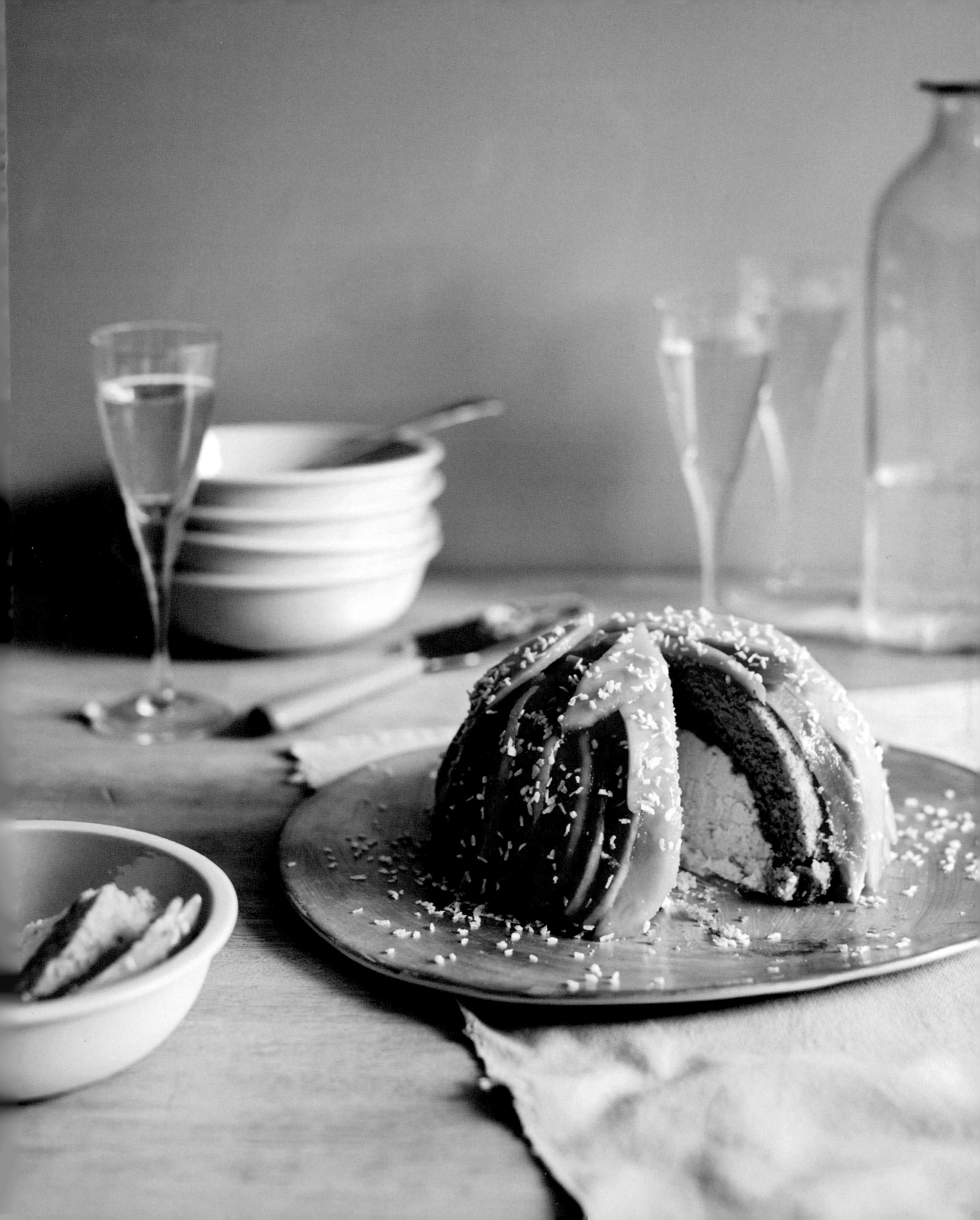

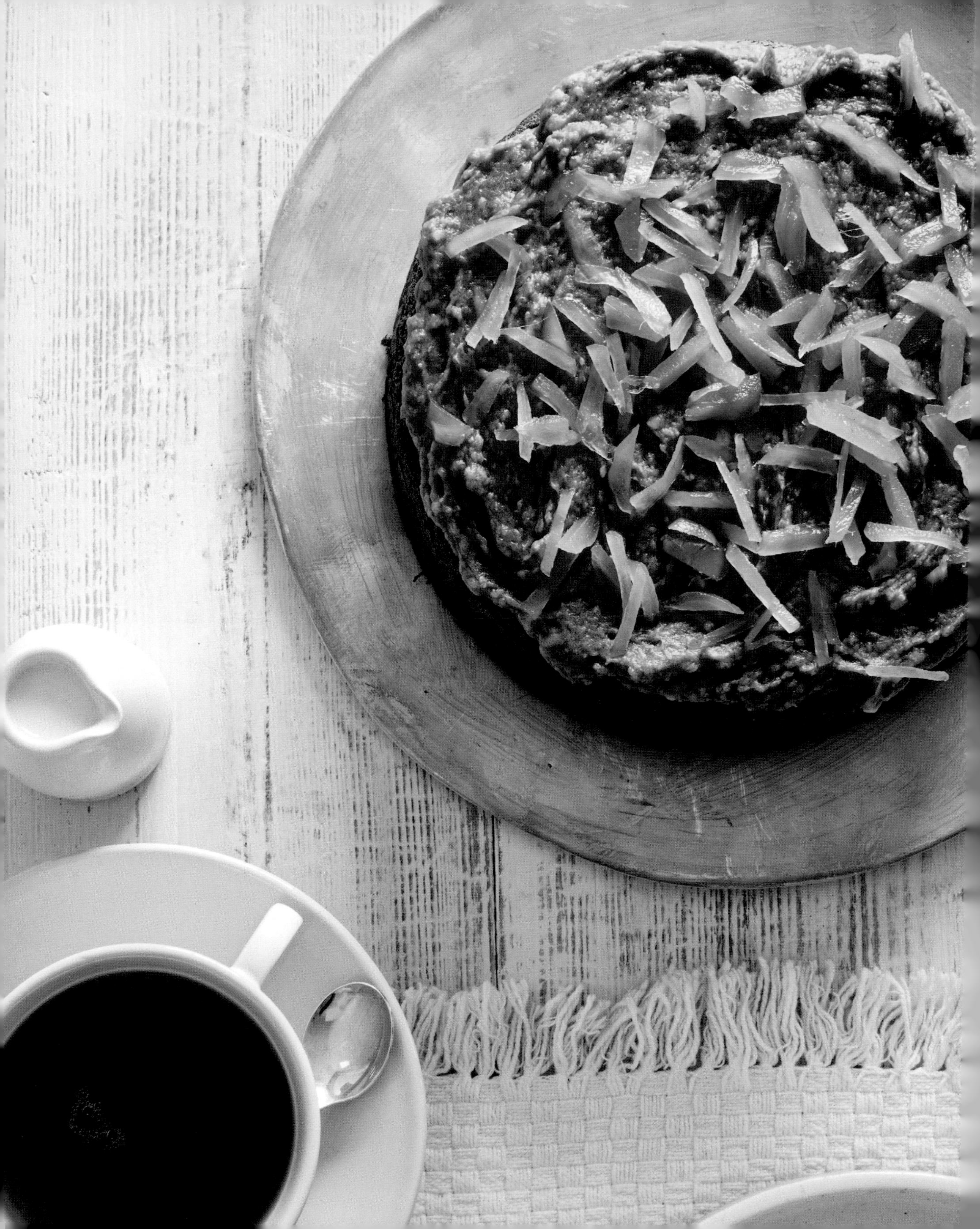

date and ginger cake

A perfect combination to go with an afternoon cup of tea on a Sunday. I made this for my sister's birthday and added vanilla crème anglaise with cooked rhubarb slices and compote. It went down well, and to my surprise the cake got better after a day or two, (not usually how cakes work). But I think it's because all the syrups and juices from the fruit really had time to soak in and settle.

7 egg yolks

5 egg whites

10 Medjool dates, stoned/pitted

200 g/2 cups ground almonds

3½ teaspoons ground ginger

1 teaspoon bicarbonate of/baking soda

6 dates, cut into pieces (I cut them into eighths)

2 teaspoons pure vanilla extract

2–3 tablespoons syrup from a jar of stem ginger

2–3 tablespoons date syrup

6 pieces of jarred stem ginger, cut into slivers, to decorate

frosting (optional)

240 g/2⅓ cups coconut butter

120 g/scant ½ cup date syrup

2 tablespoons syrup from the jar of stem ginger

2 tablespoons arrowroot

a 20-cm/8-inch round cake pan, greased and lined with baking parchment

SERVES 10

Preheat the oven to 170°C (325°F) Gas 3.

Separate the eggs in two medium mixing bowls. The yolks should go into the larger bowl if you are using different sized bowls as all the ingredients will end up in that bowl. Set aside.

In a small mixing bowl, add water (no more than 6 tablespoons) to the Medjool dates and mash to a purée. I tend to add water a couple of tablespoons at a time; it's easier to add more than take away.

In another mixing bowl, mix together the ground almonds, ground ginger and bicarbonate of/baking soda.

Add the Medjool date purée, cut dates (if using) and vanilla to the egg yolks and mix well.

Whisk the egg whites to form soft peaks.

Add the dry ingredients to the yolk and date mixture and, once everything is well combined, fold in the eggs whites. When incorporating egg whites, I tend to start with one large spoonful to loosen the mix, then carefully fold in the rest with a slotted spoon.

Pour the mixture into the prepared cake pan and bake in the preheated oven for 25–30 minutes, or until a metal skewer comes out clean. You may need to cover the top loosely with foil or baking parchment after 20 minutes of baking to stop it from colouring too much.

Warm the stem ginger syrup and date syrup together in a small saucepan over low heat. Remove the cake from the oven, lightly prick all over and brush with the warmed syrups. Cool in the cake pan on a wire rack for 10–15 minutes, then remove from the pan and leave to finish cooling.

To make the frosting, make sure the coconut butter is at room temperature so that it is soft enough to whisk. Using a handheld electric whisk, whiz the ingredients together.

Spread the frosting over the cooled cake and decorate with slivers of stem ginger to serve.

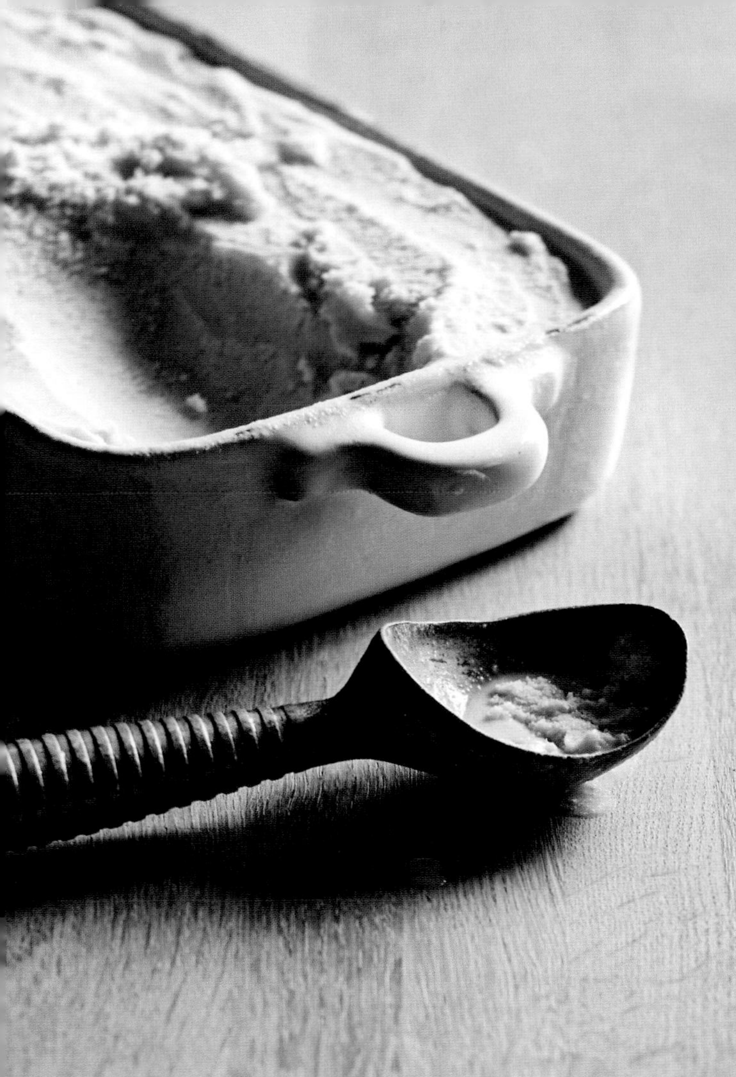

cognac ice cream

I love making this ice cream to have stashed in the freezer for ice cream emergencies. It's dairy-free and laced with Cognac for an indulgent frozen treat.

2 x 400-ml/14-oz. cans coconut milk
170 g/$^{2}/_{3}$ cup honey
4 egg yolks
50 ml/3$^{1}/_{2}$ tablespoons Cognac (make sure it's good quality, no added nonsense)

an ice-cream maker

SERVES 8–10

Put the coconut milk and honey in a saucepan over low heat. Whisk well so that it warms through evenly and the ingredients are combined.

In a metal bowl whisk the egg yolks.

Temper the yolks by slowly adding the warmed milk a little at a time, stirring continuously.

Return the mixture to the saucepan and stir constantly over low heat until it reaches a temperature of 80–85°C (105–120°F). This is to pasteurize the eggs, which is important if you are serving to those with an impaired immune system.

Transfer the mixture to a clean metal bowl and add the Cognac. Whisk well and lay a piece of clingfilm/plastic wrap over the surface so that it sits on top of the mix to stop a skin forming.

Refrigerate until completely cooled.

Churn in batches in the ice-cream maker, then store in the freezer or serve immediately.

chai tea and banana ice cream

My mum used to peel and freeze bananas and put them through our old-fashioned juicer. It used to grind and purée the fruit and come out like whipped ice cream.

2 handfuls of cashew nuts

600 ml/2 1/3 cups almond milk

5 chai tea bags

2 bananas

2 tablespoons coconut oil

4 Medjool dates

to serve

flaked or chopped nuts

desiccated/shredded coconut

ground cacao nibs

a high-powered blender (I use a NutriBullet)

an ice-cream maker

MAKES 650 ML/ 1¼ PINTS

Soak the cashews in water for at least 1 hour – the longer you soak them the easier they will be to blend.

Pour the almond milk into a saucepan and set over medium heat to warm. Remove the pan from the heat, add the tea bags and leave to infuse for at least 20 minutes.

Squeeze out the tea bags to get as much of the flavour as possible into the milk.

Strain the cashews and put in the blender with a cup of the chai-infused almond milk. Blend until smooth, then add the rest of the ingredients and blend again.

Transfer to an ice-cream maker and churn in batches, then freeze.

Remove from freezer 5–10 minutes before serving. I recommend serving with flaked or chopped nuts, desiccated/shredded coconut and cacao nibs.

Note: Buy a peppermill and fill it with cacao (or cocoa) nibs – you will get a lovely fine chocolate sprinkle.

tropical sweet potato snow

I originally wrote this recipe to go alongside a gin panna cotta with a juniper syrup, but I really enjoy it on its own. It is a good alternative to sorbet and something just a little different.

1 mango, juiced

250 ml/1 cup passion fruit juice

1/2 pineapple, juiced

2/3 tablespoon xylitol

1/3 giant sweet potato, juiced

1 egg white, lightly whisked

MAKES 300 ML/½ PINT

Pour the mango, passion fruit and pineapple juices with the xylitol into a saucepan and warm over medium heat.

Remove the pan from the heat and add the sweet potato juice and 125 ml/1/2 cup water.

Pour into an ice cream maker and, once the mixture is below 0°C add the whisked egg white.

Store in the freezer and serve in little snow cones or cups. If the snow is frozen solid, don't panic. Use a metal spoon and scrape the surface to get the snow consistency required for serving.

index

resources

Biona Organic
biona.co.uk
Organic canned or bottled products (juices, coconut cream)

Choc Chick
chocchick.com
Raw chocolate and chocolate kits

Clarks
clarksit.co.uk
Pure maple syrup and other natural sweeteners

Great Lakes
greatlakesgelatin.com
All natural gelatin

Koko® Dairy Free
kokodairyfree.com
Coconut yogurt and milk product

Manuka Wholefoods Ltd.
www.manukawholefoods.co.uk
Family-run, organic wholefood store in Chichester, UK.

NutriBullet
nutribullet.com
High-speed blenders

Planet Organic
planetorganic.com
Fully certified organic supermarket in the UK

Source at Hungerford Park
www.hungerfordpark.com/source-farm-shop
Farm store and producer.

St. Dalfour
stdalfour.co.uk
All natural jams/jellies and preserves

SunWarrior®
sunwarrior.com
All natural powders

Urban Fruit
urbanfruit.co.uk
Naturally dried fruit

Whole Foods Market
wholefoodsmarket.com
Supermarket for free-from produce

Willie's Cacao
williescacao.com
High-quality chocolate

acknowledgments

To Juliet, Milli, Holly and Ollie, I feel truly blessed to have had your support along my journey. You have each nurtured me and given me invaluable advice and amazing opportunities. You have made work so enjoyable and always kept me smiling. I admire each of you and your incredible creations in the kitchen.

Thank you to Steph, my wonderful editor, for approaching me about this book, for being on the end of the phone and responding to every email at my every need. To Sonya, for her stunning design work. Thank you to Mowie, Rachel and Jen, for capturing each dish so beautifully. It was such a pleasure to work alongside the three of you. And a big thank you to the rest of the Ryland Peters & Small team who have worked so hard behind the scenes on this book.

A heartfelt thanks to Emma and Toby (my auntie and uncle) whose organic farm has provided wonderful ingredients and inspiration for many of my recipes. Another big thank you to my very talented sister Lily, for her incredible and beautiful illustrations. Finally, to my Mum, Dad, Mike, Caroline, Jacob and Lily for their constant support throughout. I am so grateful to have such an encouraging family behind me, without you, all this would not be possible.

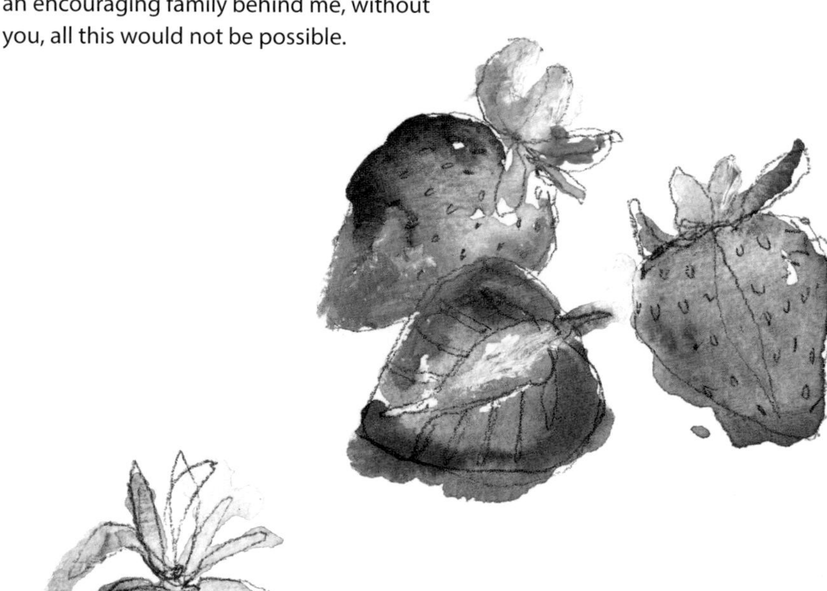

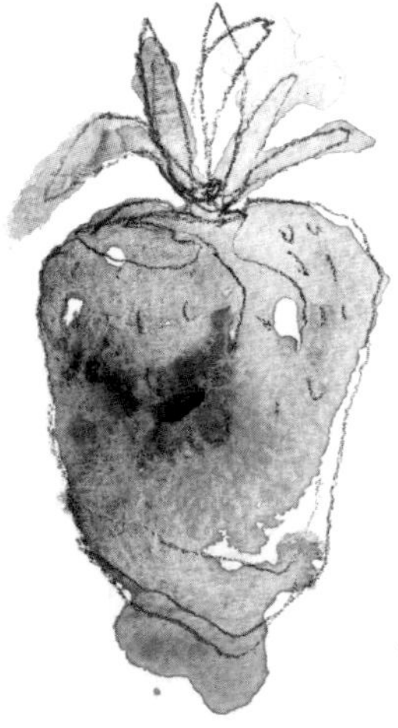

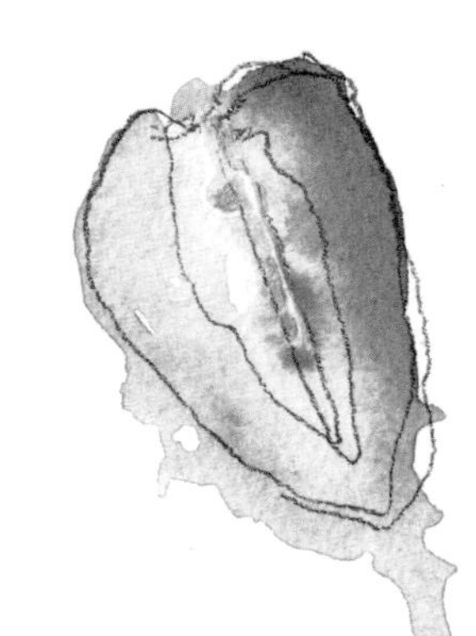

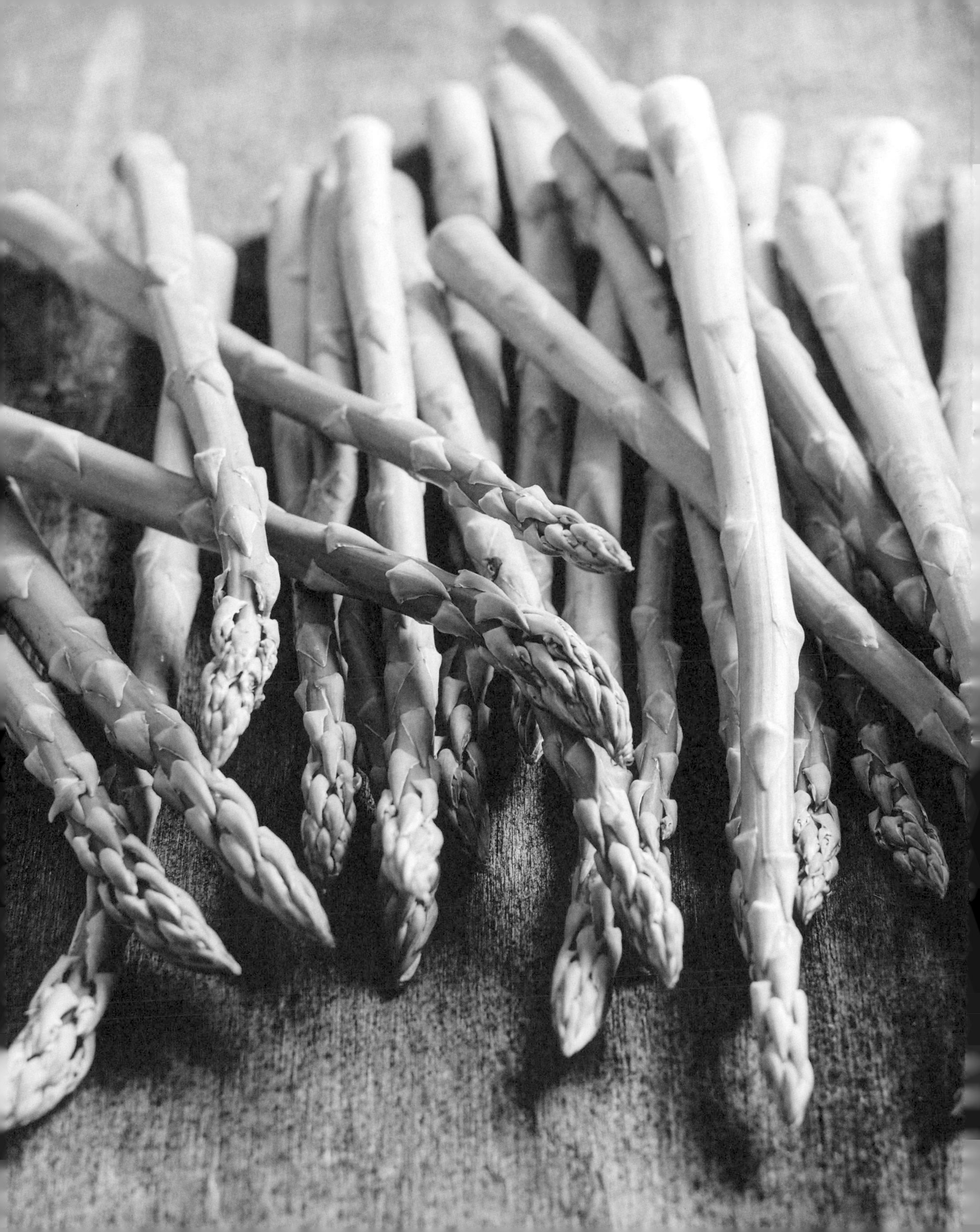